Patterns of Shock

IMPLICATIONS FOR NURSING CARE

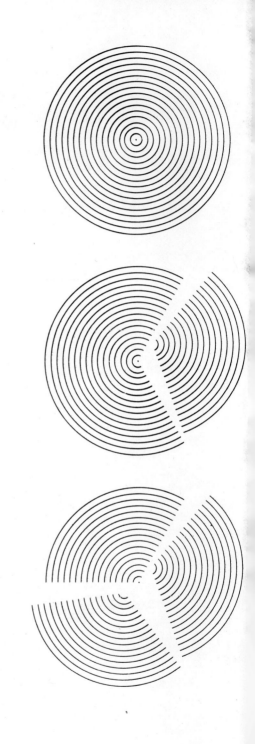

10. The amount of oxygen that can be transported by the red blood cells is directly proportionate to the quality and quantity of hemoglobin within the red cells. 33

11. Adequate circulation of blood to all body parts is dependent upon a proportionate equilibrium between the blood volume, the strength of cardiac contractions, and the size of the lumina of the blood vessels. 36

12. Anything that causes an increase in the number of red blood cells, or that decreases the plasma volume will lead to an increase in the viscosity of the blood. 39

13. There is an inverse relationship between the viscosity of the blood and the velocity of blood flow:
a. An increased viscosity leads to a decreased velocity.
b. A decreased viscosity leads to an increased velocity. 39

14. The proper functioning of all body tissues is dependent on a sufficient quality and volume of blood flowing under sufficient pressure. 39

15. An adequate cardiac output is basic to the health and proper functioning of all body tissues. 40,228

16. The heart can eject into the arterial circuit only that amount of blood it receives from the venous circuit. 40,168

17. A constant supply of blood and the removal of wastes from the myocardium are basic for adequate myocardial contractions. 40

18. There is a direct relationship between metabolic rate and cardiac rate.
a. Increased metabolism increases the heart rate.
b. Decreased metabolism decreases the heart rate. 42,230

19. The rate at which blood will flow through a blood vessel is determined by the pressure difference at each end of the vessel, the resistance to blood flow, and the viscosity of the blood. 42

20. There is a direct relationship between metabolism and carbon dioxide production; as metabolism increases, the amount of carbon dioxide produced by the tissues increases. 57

21. There is a direct relationship between metabolism and the amount of blood required by the tissues; when metabolism increases, the blood flow is correspondingly increased. 57

22. The movement of fluids from one area to another is dependent upon a difference in pressure. 66

23. Fluids flow from areas of greater to lesser points of pressure. 66

24. There is an inverse relationship between the intrathoracic pressure and the return of venous blood to the right atrium.
a. An increased intrathoracic pressure leads to a decreased return of venous blood to the right atrium.
b. A decreased intrathoracic pressure leads to an increased return of venous blood to the right atrium. 66

25. A state of health implies a dynamic equilibrium of the body and its parts; homeostasis. 74

26. Adaptation is basic to survival. 77

27. Adaptation implies protection and survival. 88

28. The extent and course of an illness are the result of the degree to which the organism fails to adapt. 88

29. Failure to adapt results in disease or death. 88

Patterns of Shock SECOND EDITION

IMPLICATIONS FOR NURSING CARE

Katherine J. Bordicks, M.S.N.

Macmillan Publishing Co., Inc.
NEW YORK

COLLIER MACMILLAN PUBLISHERS
LONDON

Macmillian Publishing Co., Inc.
866 Third Avenue, New York, New York 10022

Collier Macmillan Canada, Ltd.

Library of Congress Cataloging in Publication Data

Bordicks, Katherine J.
  Patterns of shock.

  Includes bibliographies and index.
  I. Shock. 2. Shock—Nursing. I. Title.
RB150.S5B6 1980   617'.21   79–9824
ISBN 0–02–312450–4

Printing: 1 2 3 4 5 6 7 8   Year: 0 1 2 3 4 5 6

This book is dedicated to

my students: past, present, and future

and to
my teachers and colleagues who have
inspired me

"I covet the day when practitioners will routinely theorize as they make and record their observations. When that day comes, nursing will be as committed to knowing as to doing; and the profession will have arrived."
—"On the Professional Status of Nursing", by *Rozella M. Schlotfeldt, Nursing Forum,* Vol. XIII, No. 1, 1974, pp. 16–31.

FOREWORD

This timely second edition of Katherine Bordicks' *Patterns of Shock* reaches directly to the heart of professional nursing practice. Material from the valuable previous edition has been incorporated, amplified, and rearranged in an erudite manner. The scientific information is valid, and the conclusions drawn are eminently practical.

This very readable book, written for nurses by an expert nursing practitioner makes for fascinating reading and in-depth study. The "Common Denominator Theory" as presented and identified in the text passes the realm of theory, and establishes the all-important background for effective professional nursing practice. It opens the field for investigative study, for which impressive logically arranged material is presented. Internalization of the content is facilitated by the literary skill of the author. Her dedicated, caring personality is reflected in the heart-warming focus on the patient.

Elizabeth Williams Graves
Professor Emerita
University of Mississippi,
Medical Center
Jackson, Mississippi

PREFACE TO THE SECOND EDITION

"The intellect, like an opera glass, should
only be turned up to a certain point; if
you turn it any further, you see more
hazily."
—*Leo Tolstoi*

The main purpose of this edition is to present an increased scientific base of knowledge to help nurses make judgments based on scientific facts in their care of patients. The nurse needs to be able to establish a scientific method in assessing priorities of care as patients' conditions change.

This edition introduces the reader to my Common Denominator Theory, a physiological model which represents denominators that are common to most disease conditions. In using this theory as a basis for teaching medical-surgical, maternity, pediatric, and community health nursing, students have been able to apply it in determining and giving intelligent nursing care at various levels of patient-illness. Patient progress has been noticeable.

This edition presents those materials that are necessary for the nurse to understand. I have deliberately omitted details I believe to be irrelevent to the teaching and practice of nursing.

More clinical examples have been added to facilitate the understanding of additional conditions that can cause shock. It is hoped that this book will serve as a model for students, nurse practitioners, and nurse educators.

Katherine J. Bordicks
New Orleans, Louisiana

"Teaching, always new, always dynamic, always wonderful, means channeling students' vision to reason while holding them firm in the conviction that there is nothing to fear from reason, that therein lies its strength."*

---

* Mae Venable: "What Teaching Means to Me," *Davis' Nursing Survey,* Vo. XXIII, No. 5, Oct., 1959, F. A. Davis Co., Medical Publishers, Phila., p. 149.

PREFACE TO THE FIRST EDITION

"He only can be said to be the doer of
a thing, that hath the will and the knowledge in the doing it."
—*Lactantius*

This is a book on shock—it includes the physiologic patterns of major shock conditions that are encountered very often in the practice of nursing. Shock can occur in any hospital area—medical, surgical, orthopedic, obstetric, operating and recovery rooms, psychiatry, dermatology, metabolic, and so on. Shock can occur in any home, on any street, in any doctor's or dentist's office. In a word, shock can occur anywhere. Sometimes shock occurs when it could have and should have been prevented.

Knowledge and understanding of scientific principles are basic to intelligent nursing care of patients suffering from any of the various types of shock. Although the signs and symptoms exhibited by patients in different types of shock are similar, the nursing care implications can be quite different. For example, patients in vasogenic shock and patients in hemorrhagic shock have similar signs and symptoms; but if the treatment and nursing care for the patient in hemorrhagic shock were administered to the patient in vasogenic shock (or vice versa), the results could prove disastrous.

While much has been written about shock in the medical literature, the technical terminology and the omission of relevant basic anatomy and physiology often fail to give the nurse a clear picture from
which she can draw implications for individualized nursing care. Without such a background of understanding, there may be a tendency
to apply the same nursing care to all patients suffering from different
types of shock. Therefore, I have included many pertinent basic scientific elements in order that the nurse may more fully comprehend
the scientific implications for nursing care of these patients. This, to
my knowledge, has not been done before.

I believe that a subject can be understood only when the components of the subject are understood; otherwise, true learning and subsequent intelligent nursing practice cannot possibly take place. Like the
pieces of a jigsaw puzzle, the pieces of knowledge must be sorted
carefully and fitted together properly, or a meaningful picture will
not result. The purpose of this book, then, is to present those pieces
of knowledge that are involved in understanding the various types
of shock, to sort them, to fit them together, and it is hoped, to emerge,
with true pictures of shock which the nurse needs to understand before
she can give intelligent and purposeful nursing care.

Presently we are engaged in a crucial era of nursing. On one
side of the fence we hear some leaders' voices asserting, "The nurse
must be more prepared to assume an administrative role." On the
other side of the fence, another faction of nursing leaders is pleading,
"Put the registered nurse back at the patient's bedside!" While all
along, the clinical nurse practitioner is tottering on top of the fence;
she is confused as to what she *should* be doing; she is placed in a
double bind!

Be that as it may, whichever role she is to assume, the nurse
needs an intelligent grounding in the arts and sciences pertinent to
the clinical practice of nursing. Without these, how could she possibly
be an effective administrator—for does she not have to know, understand, and possess the ability to apply the constituents of nursing care
if she is to guide the nursing activities of others, or if she herself is
to give effective bedside nursing care? In a word, inadequate preparation in theory and practice can only lead to inadequate administrative
functions.

Regardless of the two opposing points of view of present nursing
leaders, there is one point on which they agree—the necessity for a
meaningful education which will equip the nurse to function intelli-

gently in the clinical setting, be she nurse administrator or bedside nurse. The over-all goal of any nurse must be the same: to assist the patient to a state of optimum health. Ours is not to add to his ills through ignorant or sympathetic neglect, nor is it to impose iatrogenic diseases upon him. It has been said, "You have to be more than just a nice guy; you have to be the captain."

We who are engaged in education often lose sight of our main reason for being—to prepare nurses for the realistic practice of nursing. And so it follows that we lose sight of just what it is we are trying to teach, and why. Unless we keep our main purpose before us in constant view, we are inclined to pour into the students' minds a confluence of unrelated and unnecessary facts—facts which, isolated as they are so often, tend only to produce confusion, frustration, and disinterest in the students. If I may indulge in an analogy: A good cake does not just happen. The ingredients must be measured carefully and separately. Then they must be blended slowly and appropriately. After baking for a certain period of time in an oven of the right temperature, a beautiful and tasty cake will evolve. On the other hand, haphazard measurement of the ingredients, careless blending, and an oven that is either too hot or too cool will yield something other than a fine cake. Is it not the same with curriculum construction and teaching— with the student and learning?

The effective nurse practitioner must, of expedience, go through a lengthy and difficult learning process. Because human lives depend on her for their continued existence, the nurse practitioner is obligated to learn. Furthermore, the nursing profession is her choice, so she must motivate herself to learn. A phrase, unfortunately, which is often heard and reiterated by nurse educators is, "We must motivate the student to learn." I wholeheartedly agree with Charlotte Towle, who opposes this point of view:

> Traditionally, educators have been concerned to motivate the learner. For productive outcomes in learning, they have sought to stimulate active interest in a field of study through appeal to associated interests and by other special devices. This responsibility to foster interest is appropriately assumed at the lower educational levels where students are required to attend school. In professional education the educator does not have the same responsibility to incite interest. If the field of study does not progressively engage the learner, it may well be that he belongs elsewhere. It is possible, however, for an educational regime to obstruct learning. Through needlessly creating stress, it may lead to automatic,

rather than creative effort, fragmentation rather than integration, and hence to a breakdown in drives originally appropriate and strong."*

This era of nursing is quite different from any other, and the next era will be different from the present one. Yet, the basic scientific principles are the same, and they will remain the same. Additional discoveries in science will be made, and, when they are, we must accept them and adapt them to the nursing care of our patients. How else can we justify our continued existence as a profession?

In its own small way, it is hoped that this book will be practical, and therefore useful, for the student nurse, practitioner, educator, and administrator of nursing.

Katherine J. Bordicks

---

* Charlotte Towle: *The Learner in Education for the Professions*, (Chicago: University of Chicago Press, 1954), p. 134.

ACKNOWLEDGMENTS

I am deeply grateful to Doctor Faustena Blaisdell, Mrs. Elizabeth W. Graves, Miss Eleanor A. Callahan, and Miss Nancy McCain, who read the entire manuscript of this book and offered valuable suggestions to enhance its clarity. Their support and encouragement during this huge task will never be forgotten.

I wish also to express my sincere gratitude to my following colleagues and friends for their suggestions pertaining to various sections of the book: Mrs. Bobbie G. Ward, Miss Rene M. Reeb, Mrs. Kay Milhorn, Mrs. Marilyn Wenzel, and Dr. Elizabeth S. Martin.

K. J. B.

CONTENTS

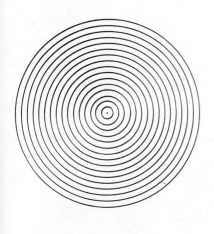

PART I

A Scientific Background Basic to the Understanding of Shock

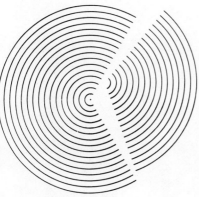

The simple and elementary is always conceivable without the complex, whereas the complex cannot be conceived of without the elementary.
—*Ivan Pavlov*

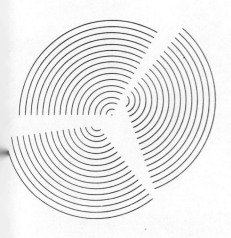

CHAPTER 1

In Search of a Theory for Nursing

"The focus of any profession's scientific
concern is interdependent with the profession's service; its social function."
—*Dorothy E. Johnson*[1]

"If you give a man a fish he will have a single meal. If you teach him *how*
to fish, he will eat for the rest of his life."
—*A Chinese Proverb*

To learn structure is to learn how things are related. Nurses should
be educated to learn underlying structures which will enable them
to get a general understanding of the subject matter.

Scientifically supported generalizations and nursing research
must form the basis of a theoretical model of nursing practice. Without
this base, nursing can only be practiced by intuition. In her excellent
and classic article, Faye McCain has stated

Patient assessment is the responsibility of the professional nurse. When
professional nurses are more knowledgeable in the contributory sciences,
and become more competent in analytical thinking, some of these judgments probably will be independent judgments upon which nurses will
make decisions without waiting for medical direction. Professional nurses

---

[1] Dorothy E. Johnson, "Development of Theory: A Requisite for Nursing as a Primary
Health Profession," *Nursing Research*, 23 (Sept.–Oct. 1974), 373.

can, do, and should make judgments. . . . Nursing, as it is taught and practiced today, is primarily intuitive. However, the need for a precise method has been recognized.[2]

A theory has a very specific meaning; it consists of a group of generalizations which are deductively connected. Nurse educators are greatly concerned with the structure and content of curricula. This concern, according to Styles, is because "the nursing profession lacks coherence; that is, the quality of being logically integrated, consistent, and intelligible."[3] Nursing educators are beginning to realize that an approach to nursing education is needed that focuses on generalizations that apply to *many* patients, regardless of their diagnoses.

According to Torres, content should include materials that are representative of the field as a whole. A relatively small volume of knowledge may be sufficient for the understanding of a larger body of material. She points out that "this approach is essential today, with the vast proliferation of knowledge and can be best achieved by utilizing key concepts."[4] The desire today is to develop students who can *think,* and who can apply their knowledge in many situations. Memorization of isolated facts is *not* implicit in learning.

MacDowell and Jones state that "nurse educators must find a way to meaningfully prepare future nurses, elucidating new theories, making the complex simple, establishing the heart of the matter so that the body is not treated separately from the mind, the spirit not separated from the body and mind, and parts of the body not separated from the whole.[5]

Over the years, Masters students have told me that they would like to elect medical-surgical nursing as their clinical major, "but," they said, "there are just too many disease conditions." True, in comparison with other major areas, medical-surgical nursing is inclusive of a vaster territory. I began to think that there *must* be some common features which are applicable to most, if not all, disease conditions. From this has evolved what I call my Common Denominator Theory.

[2] Faye McCain, "Nursing by Assessment—Not Intuition," *American Journal of Nursing* (April 1965), 83–84.
[3] Margretta M. Styles, "Continuing Education in Nursing: One Hope for Professional Coherence," *Nurse Educator,* 1 (July–Aug. 1976), 6–9.
[4] Gertrude Torres, "Unifying the Curriculum—The Integrated Approach," New York: *National League for Nursing,* 1974.
[5] Mary Beth McDowell, and Cynthia Jones, *An Analysis of the Pathophysiology of Selected Diseases to Document Katherine J. Bordicks' Common Denominator Theory,* unpublished study, Masters Program in Nursing, The University of Mississippi, Aug. 1976, p. 3.

I have used this theory for five years, always sharing with my students that while it may not be all-inclusive, at least it is a start. Their acceptance and use of this theory has been very gratifying. It has provided them with an underlying structure which has facilitated their understanding of the relationships between the parts and the whole.

In the summer of 1976, two of my students did a mini library-search to determine the applicability of the Common Denominator Theory. They studied thirty different disease conditions and found that the theory was applicable to all thirty conditions. In their review of the literature, McDowell and Jones state, "Nothing was found that identified common pathophysiology of diseases that nurses could use to facilitate their understanding of how diseases affect individuals. However, the Common Denominator Theory offers fulfillment of this need."[6]

The Common Denominator Theory: A Physiological Model

In the Common Denominator Theory, it is theorized that there are certain significant physiological features that occur in most (all?) disease conditions.* These are:

1. Disease is a stressor which elicits the General Adaptation Syndrome (G.A.S.), a generalized neuro-hormonal compensatory response.
2. Disease affects the homeostasis of the whole body, including cells, tissues, organs, and systems.
3. Disease affects the normal metabolism (increased or decreased functioning) of one or more of the four types of body cells, namely, muscle, nerve, connective, and epithelial.
4. Disease alters the supply (increased or decreased) of one or more of the five substances needed by the cells, tissues, organs, and systems, namely, oxygen, nutrients, water, electrolytes, and hormones. There is an alteration in the removal of cell wastes.
5. Disease leads to a disproportion of fluid and electrolytes between the three fluid compartments of the body, namely, intravascular, interstitial, and intracellular compartments.

[6] Ibid, p. 10.
* Diseases of physical or psychological origin.

The preceding represents a core of knowledge from which an understanding of disease states and scientific implications for nursing care can be drawn. It is first requisite, however, that there be broad, general knowledge of *normal* physiology, before the abnormal, or altered physiological state with its ramifications and implications can be comprehended.

Probably the most gratifying feature of this theory is that the learners will discover that it is no longer necessary to memorize signs and symptoms; they should be able to *think* them through. Is *this* not the meaning of education?

All of the identified common denominators apply to shock, as well as to other diseases. The section on shock will be used as a model which exemplifies this theory. The basic scientific background materials which are presented in this book are inclusive of materials which exemplify the Common Denominator Theory.

REFERENCES

Brodbeck, May. "The Philosophy of Science and Educational Research." *Review of Educational Research,* 28 (Dec. 1957), 427–440.

Bruner, Jerome S. *The Process of Education.* New York: Vintage Books, 1960.

Palmer, Mary Ellen. "Patient-Centered Problems Approach to Teaching Medical-Surgical Nursing." *Nursing Outlook,* 9 (July 1961), 411–413.

Reilly, Dorothy E. "Why a Conceptual Framework?" *Nursing Outlook,* 23 (Sept. 1975), 567.

CHAPTER 2

An Introduction to Shock

Shock, due to any cause, represents circulatory failure with all of its ramifications. The complications and mortality rate caused by shock are high. In many instances, prompt recognition and treatment of early circulatory failure can prevent the development of severe shock, thereby decreasing the incidence of complications and death.

The patient suffering from any type of shock requires immediate and intelligent nursing attention. Although accurate observation and reporting of signs and symptoms are extremely important components of the nurse's duties, something further is required of the nurse—intelligent action. This implies an understanding of the scientific principles involved in the individual patient situation, or else the nurse may be too late to save a life.

"Shock," per se, is not a disease; but rather, it is an untoward effect of many different disease conditions. Some authorities have urged that the term "shock" be discarded, because there is no such thing as the treatment of "shock"; but rather only the treatment of the patient *in shock* due to a primary disease. In a strict sense, shock is a feature of *all* terminal illnesses, for, in the final analysis, everyone dies in a state of shock.

The etiologies of shock are numerous; this is what makes it a difficult and perplexing study. Consider, for example, the certainty that all cases of tuberculosis are caused by the *same* organism, the Mycobacterium tuberculosis. All cases of diphtheria are caused by the same organism, Corynebacterium diphtheriae. If all shock conditions resulted from a single cause, the nursing and medical management of patients would be less puzzling and more expeditious. For instance, suppose a city could be attacked from any one of seven roads leading to it. Unless the enemy is sighted, the soldiers of the city may take up arms of defense against an empty road—valiantly, but uselessly. And so the city will be overwhelmed by the enemy. But if only one road led to the city, adequate defense could be assured.

Shock affects the *whole* body; it affects the metabolism of every cell, tissue, organ, and system. Hence, it will be expedient to discuss some of the basic aspects of normal structure and function. Unless the normal pattern is understood, there will be little to no understanding of the abnormal and its untoward implications. When the nurse has an understanding of the basic processes that keep the body in a state of healthy equilibrium, she will be disinclined to memorize signs and symptoms of each disease entity. Instead, she will discover commonalities of disease conditions. At the point where she begins to understand the basic physiological ramifications, she will begin to observe and perceive the patient in greater scientific depth. Knowing what to look for, she will be observant for beginning appearances of signs and symptoms, rather than wait until they have become full-blown.

Definition of Shock

Shock is an abnormal physiological state characterized by a disproportion between the circulating blood volume and the size of the vascular bed, resulting in circulatory failure and tissue hypoxia. "Shock" is a descriptive term denoting a syndrome characterized by protracted prostration and hypotension. It is now widely agreed that tissue perfusion is of greater importance than maintaining the arterial blood pressure. Usually, shock is accompanied by pallor, cool and moist skin, collapse of superficial veins, alterations in mental status, and suppression of the formation of urine.

CAUSES OF SHOCK

The three causes of shock are:

Decreased blood volume
Failure of the heart
Increased peripheral vasodilatation

All conditions leading to shock fall into one, or a combination of these three causes.

Correlated with the Common Denominator Theory:

1. Shock represents a severe stressor which imposes a powerful neuro-endocrine reaction (the G.A.S.) on the body, which is compensatory in nature; unless the patient is treated, compensatory failure will ensue.
2. Shock affects the homeostasis of all body parts: muscle, nerve, connective, and epithelial cells; and, since cells form the basis for tissues, organs, systems, and the whole organism, these likewise are affected. From these, signs and symptoms derive.
3. and 4. Shock leads to a decreased supply of the five substances needed for cell health and metabolism, namely, oxygen, nutrients, water, electrolytes, and hormones.
5. Shock leads to a disproportion of fluid and electrolytes between the three fluid compartments of the body.

The opposite of shock is a state of health, which implies that the volume of blood, the cardiac muscle pump action, and the size of the vascular bed are in a state of dynamic equilibrium; therefore, all parts of the body receive the amount of blood needed to sustain circulatory health. Each of these components can undergo considerable alteration and still support an adequate circulation of blood, as long as the compensatory alterations of the other two components are maintained satisfactorily. Shock occurs when an effective combination of this triad of components cannot be maintained. Circulatory failure results from a deficiency of any one, two, or all three components.

A CLASSIFICATION OF SHOCK

Shock can be classified in many different ways. However, since shock is due to the failure of any one of these three components, i.e., blood volume, cardiac muscle pump, or vascular dilatation, the

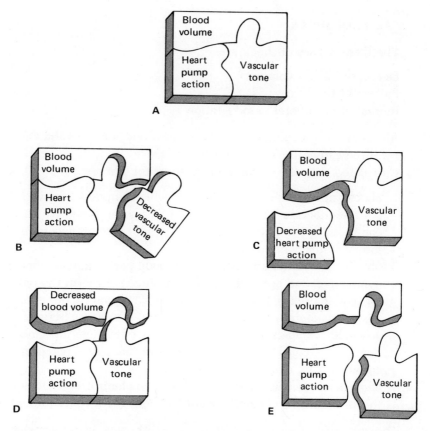

Figure 1. A. *Circulatory homeostasis—dynamic equilibrium established by blood volume, heart pump action, and vascular tone.*

B. *Decreased vascular tone—vasodilatation.*

C. *Decreased heart pump action—cardiac failure.*

D. *Decreased blood volume—hemorrhage, plasma and/or electrolyte loss.*

E. *Shock—a disproportion between the circulating blood volume and the size of the vascular bed.*

most logical classification to use is the one proposed by Blalock based upon these three dominant physiological mechanisms.

Blood volume (hypovolemic shock)

Synonyms: Hematogenic Shock, Oligemic Shock.

Hypovolemic shock represents a reduction in blood volume, due to a decrease in whole blood or plasma. Examples to be discussed in this book are:

1. Hemorrhagic shock
2. Burn shock
3. Traumatic shock, including fractures
4. Diabetic shock
5. Bowel obstruction.

Cardiac muscle pump (normovolemic shock)
Cardiogenic shock represents failure of the heart to pump the blood. To be discussed: shock caused by left heart failure.

Vascular tone
Vasogenic and neurogenic shock are characterized by profound peripheral vasodilatation. To be discussed:

1. Spinal anaesthesia shock
2. Insulin shock
3. Anaphylactic shock
4. Septic shock, toxic shock.

Other
A decreased cardiac output can result from any condition that decreases the venous return to the right side of the heart, even though the blood volume, heart pump, and vascular tone are in a state of dynamic equilibrium. To be discussed:

1. The Valsalva maneuver
2. Paradoxical respirations, resulting from rib fractures
3. Mediastinal shift, due to pneumothorax.

CHAPTER 3

The Structural and Functional Pattern of the Body

Basic to the understanding of shock is an understanding of the fundamentals involved in it. A builder always starts from a foundation and builds upward—at least I have never heard of one who can start building from the top. And so it should be with the teaching-learning process. Understanding fundamentals makes any subject more comprehensible.

The mastery of fundamental ideas permits an individual to grasp general principles and to develop an attitude toward learning and inquiry which can enable him to solve problems on his own. Mastery of fundamentals pays off in dividends, as he will have learned not only a specific component, but he will also have learned a model for the understanding of other components related to it. In this instance, he will have learned fundamental knowledge which is basic to many, if not all, disease conditions.

The Body as a System

"Change begets change, and change in any part creates change in the whole."—Martha E. Rogers[1]

SYSTEM

Definition: A totality of elements in mutual interaction with each other. Systems analysis is an attempt to understand a complex whole by examining its parts.

The body is an open system whose parts are mutually interconnected, interacting, and interdependent. Anything that affects the health (homeostasis) of any part of the body will affect all of its parts. The survival of a system is dependent upon the healthy interaction of its parts. Since all body systems are interrelated, the ramifications and implications of disease are reflected in them.

Body structure and function are hierarchically organized. Any disorder of the cells will affect the functioning of tissues, organs, systems, and whole body.

A system, which is a patterned form of existence, is predictable. For example, failure of a diabetic to take insulin will result in a decreased supply of glucose to body cells. As a result, the cells will not generate energy and normal cell functioning will cease. Subsequently,

[1] Martha, E. Rogers, *An Introduction to the Theoretical Basis of Nursing,* Philadelphia: F. A. Davis Co., 1970, p. 51.

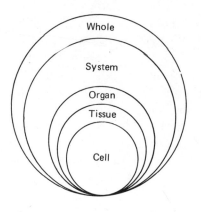

Figure 2. *The body hierarchy of structure.*

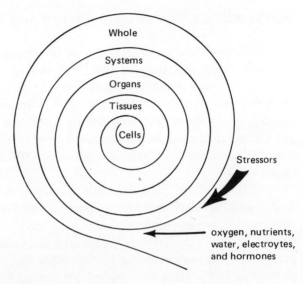

Figure 3. *The body as a system: interconnected, interacting, and interdependent.*

weakness will occur in his tissues, organs, and body systems. A collapse of the whole individual is inevitable, unless insulin is administered.

PRINCIPLE 1: While living systems can adapt to their environment, they also affect their environments and change them.

Anyone can appreciate the overall magnificence of the human body, yet something more is required of the nurse—she must understand the relationship of the parts to each other and to the whole organism. It is in the study of the human body that one becomes cognizant that the *whole* is greater than the sum of its parts. The parts and mechanisms at work within the body to keep it alive are numerous. But, knowledge, and even understanding of each distinct part, do not predispose to an understanding of the *whole* functioning organism. Understanding evolves when the pieces of knowledge are sorted and fitted together properly, so that the learner can see the relationship of one part to another part and to the whole organism.

The parts and mechanisms involved in shock are numerous. Therefore, it is essential to include sufficient and appropriate basic discussion of these parts, so that relationships can be seen, understood, and appreciated.

15

Independence Versus Dependence and Interdependence

A true state of human independence never exists. At first, one is inclined to think that it does. But think it over. If the ill person is a dependent being, does this suggest that the well person is independent? Or is the well person only less dependent? Probably the latter is more correct. The greater our need for anything, the more dependent we are. Or, we might say, increasing needs lead to increasing dependence. Patients are unable to perform the necessary homeostatic functions unaided.

Although body cells are basic, dynamic units of structure, their health and life at all times are dependent on extracellular forces. The cells, tissues, organs, and systems of each individual can carry on their normal functions *only* if they are healthy and exist in a healthy environment; this implies receiving the supplies they need. In a word, all persons and all parts of their bodies are dependent and interdependent upon other internal and external forces.

Although body cells, tissues, organs, systems, and individuals are dependent on certain materials to perform their functions, each has a *unique use* for these materials. Have we not (in our culture) placed the emphasis on the dependency and supply factors, rather than on the unique creations that can *evolve* from these supplies? Muscle, nerve, connective, and epithelial cells receive the same supplies; but they each carry out distinctively different and unique functions. An artist may be furnished with canvas and paints; a musician may be furnished a book of concertos. The important factor is the unique creations they make of these supplies.

It has been established that all living things depend on a source of supplies in order to carry out their unique functions. Dependency seems to be a law of nature; the more limited are our supplies, the greater is our dependence.

Basic Functions of the Body

One of the basic characteristics of living organisms is the ability to transform nutrients into energy. Other characteristics are:

The ability to react to stimuli
The ability to transmit impulses

The ability to move
The ability to grow
The ability to reproduce.

Units of the Body

In all types of shock, the integrity and life of body cells are threatened. Therefore, it is necessary to discuss some of the important aspects of the individual cell and its environment. First, let us consider the whole body:

Body—composed of systems, organs, tissues, and cells
Systems—composed of organs, tissues, and cells
Organs—composed of tissues and cells
Tissues—composed of cells
Cells—smallest units. Reactons and organelles are thought to be small units within the cells.

Types of Cells

Cellular homeostasis is dependent on an adequate supply of oxygen, nutrients, water, electrolytes, and hormones, an optimum temperature range, and a pH in the range of 7.35 to 7.45. Each human being is composed of about 100 trillion cells of only four different types, each with its unique bodily function. These are

1. Muscle cells. These cells form muscle tissue which possesses the ability to contract and expand. Following are the three kinds of muscle tissue:
   a. Skeletal muscle—provides power of movement and is under voluntary control.
   b. Smooth muscle—found in various visceral organs, i.e., alimentary canal, genitourinary tract, respiratory passages, and the middle layer of blood vessels. Smooth muscle is under involuntary control of the sympathetic nervous system.
   c. Cardiac muscle—these cells form the muscle tissue of the heart, the myocardium, which provides the pumping power. Cardiac muscle is under involuntary control.

17

2. Nerve cells. Bundles of nerve cells, or neurons, comprise the nerves of the body and the nerve pathways in the brain and spinal cord. Nerves possess the property of irritability and are responsible for the conduction of impulses throughout the body.

3. Connective cells. These cells form tissues that serve as binding and supportive materials; they form the framework of various organs and connect them to other body structures. Fibrous tissues, cartilage, and bone are examples of this tissue.

4. Epithelial cells. These cells form tissues that cover the surface of the body (the skin), line cavities and blood vessels (membranes), and organize into secreting organs (glands).

THE NATURE OF THE CELL AND ITS ENVIRONMENT

Within certain limits, cells can adapt to unfavorable conditions through atrophy, hypertrophy, hyperplasia, or metaplasia. All cells contain protoplasm, which is a viscous fluid consisting mainly of protein and water. The nucleus, located in the central part of the cell, is surrounded by its own membrane. Apparently the protoplasm is dependent on, and regulated by the nucleus, for if the nucleus is removed, the cell will die.

With the exception of urine and bile, all body cells and all body fluids contain protein.

THE PERMEABILITY OF THE CELL MEMBRANE

The cell wall is an extremely thin membrane which serves as a protection against invaders, but also permits water, oxygen, nutrients, electrolytes, and some hormones to enter it, thus providing for cellular sustenance and the creation of energy. The membrane also allows waste products to leave the cell by the process of diffusion.

The semipermeable cell membrane is selectively permeable; this means that while it permits some substances to enter the cell, it does not permit others to do so. Whether or not molecules can pass through the cell membrane is determined by the following factors:

1. The size of the molecules. Small molecules can enter the cell more readily than large molecules. However, large fat-soluble molecules can enter the cell while large protein molecules cannot.

2. Electrical charges. In some instances, the electrical charges present on cell surfaces are important in determining whether a substance can be admitted to the cell. For example, the red blood cell has a positively charged membrane; therefore, positively charged substances outside the red cell are repelled, and their entrance into it is barred. Negatively charged and uncharged ions, on the other hand, can enter readily, and, simultaneously, an equal number of negatively charged and uncharged ions leave the cell.

PASSAGE OF SUBSTANCES ACROSS CELL MEMBRANES

The passage of substances through membranes can occur in at least four ways: by osmosis, diffusion, filtration, and secretion.

Osmosis

When two solutions of different concentrations are separated by a semipermeable membrane, the solvent of the less concentrated solution will move across the membrane into the more concentrated solution. Osmotic pressure is the pulling force exerted by the osmotic process. Since dissolved substances do not pass through the membrane, the only way for the concentration to be equalized on both sides of the membrane is for water to pass from the less concentrated to the more highly concentrated solution. Sodium and protein are great attractors of water. The protein of the plasma makes up the colloid osmotic pressure within the intravascular compartment, hence attracting water from the interstitial compartment. Sodium is another attractor of water. Although the cell membrane is permeable to water and oxygen, it is relatively impermeable to salts. If the cell is placed in a hypertonic salt solution—meaning a salt solution of greater concentration than the salt solution within the cell, water will pass out of the cell through the cell membrane by the process of osmosis, and the cell will shrink (crenation). If the cell is placed in a hypotonic solution—a concentration that is less than the salt solution within the cell—water will pass into the cell by the process of osmosis, and the cell will swell and increase in size. If not checked, the cell will burst; this is called hemolysis. Therefore, in order to maintain the normal size and subsequent normal functioning-power of the cell, the environment outside the cell (the interstitial compartment for the tissue cells, and the plasma for the red blood cells) must consist of a proper salt solution—an isotonic

19

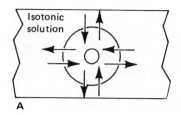

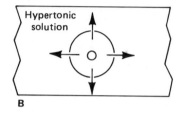

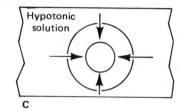

Figure 4. *Effects of fluid environment on the cell.*
    A. *Normal isotonic environment. Normal size of cell.*
    B. *Abnormal hypertonic environment. Shrinkage (crenation)*
of cell occurs.
    C. *Abnormal hypotonic environment. Swelling and eventual*
hemolysis of the cell occur.

solution—so that a proper osmotic relationship exists between the extracellular and intracellular compartments. It should be remembered that only those substances which fail to pass through the pores of a semipermeable membrane exert an osmotic pressure.

Diffusion

Diffusion refers to the movement of ions from areas of high molecular concentration to areas of lower concentration. Or, we might say that diffusion is the spreading or scattering of molecules of gases or liquids until all areas of the concentration are equalized. To cite a common example: When perfume is sprayed in a room, the perfume molecules move from the area where it is more highly concentrated to all other parts of the room. Thus the movement is in the direction of higher to lower areas of perfume-concentration, until the molecules in the room are evenly dispersed. The movement of smoke is another example of diffusion.

Since diffusion is due to the movement of molecules, any factor that increases the motion of the molecules will increase diffusion. Heat and stirring are good examples of this. Diffusion can also occur across a permeable membrane, i.e., a membrane which permits the passage of dissolved molecules. Proteins are the only dissolved substances in the plasma which do not diffuse readily from the intravascular compartment into the interstitial compartment. As a result, the protein concentration of the plasma is approximately five times that of the interstitial compartment (see Colloid Osmotic Pressure, pp. 25, 39, 52).

Filtration pressure (synonym: hydrostatic pressure)

In a container of water, the pressure on the surface of the water is equal to the atmospheric pressure. For each 13.6 mm. distance below the surface of the water, the pressure increases 1 mm. Hg. This is the result of the weight of the water, and is called hydrostatic, or filtration pressure.

In the body, filtration pressure exists when water and dissolved substances are forced through a permeable membrane from an area of higher pressure to an area of lower pressure. (Do not confuse "pressure" with "concentration".) The mechanical force responsible for this action is exerted by the pumping action of the heart. Two excellent examples of filtration occurring in the body are (1) glomerular filtration pressure, and (2) filtration at the capillary level. Filtration occurs in most of the capillaries, where capillary blood pressure forces a virtually protein-free plasma filtrate into the interstitial compartment. The fluid which passes through the capillary membrane consists of water, small proteins, and any dissolved substances of electrolytes and crystalloids to which the membrane is permeable.

Secretion

The process whereby a hormone is formed and expressed by a gland is called "secretion." The transfer of hormones across cell membranes is not clearly understood. However, it is presumed that a substance known as cyclic AMP (adenosine monophosphate), discovered by Sutherland, is necessary in the regulation of cell metabolism. That is, cyclic AMP is regarded as a second messenger necessary for hormonal regulation of intracellular metabolism.

The Milieu of the Cells: Fluid and Electrolytes

To most nurses the study of body fluids and electrolytes is most difficult. More details than the nurse needs to know in the practice of nursing tend only to confuse her. For this reason, the following materials will deal only with those aspects that will be useful to the nurse in her observation and care of patients.

Homeostasis (to be discussed in greater detail later) means a constancy of the internal milieu. The extracellular fluid and electrolytes is often called the internal environment, or the internal milieu of the body. Among other things, the homeostasis of the body implies a dynamic equilibrium of body fluids and electrolytes within the three fluid compartments of the body. Shock, on the other hand, implies an imbalance of body fluids and electrolytes, hence, an upset of the body's homeostatic equilibrium.

Normally, fluids and electrolytes are obtained from water and foods that are ingested and then absorbed into the blood stream from the gastrointestinal tract by the processes of diffusion and osmosis. The heart then pumps the blood through the blood vessels to all parts of the body. Through the processes of diffusion, filtration, and osmosis, water, nutrients, electrolytes, oxygen, and hormones are delivered to the interstitial and intracellular compartments. Through the processes of diffusion and osmosis, metabolites are removed from the cells, and enter the interstitial and intravascular compartments, respectively.

BODY FLUIDS

Pure water does not exist in the human body; it is always in combination with electrolytes. Body fluids have two overall functions: (1) to provide a medium of transport of substances from one part of the body to another, and (2) to provide an intracellular medium in which chemical reactions of the cells can occur.

AMOUNT OF WATER IN THE BODY

There is a significant difference in mean body water content between males and females, which appears at puberty and persists throughout the life span. This difference is due mainly to the amount of body fat. Since fat is essentially free of water, a thin person will contain more fluid per pound of weight than a fat person. Too, since women are composed of more fat than men, their bodies contain less water than those of men. The greatest amount of water in proportion to the per cent of body weight is in the infant.

With progressive age, body water content decreases. The total amount of water in a man of average weight is about forty liters, averaging about 57 per cent of his total body weight. (In the new born, the amount of water may be as high as 75 per cent of the body weight.) Approximately twenty-five of the forty liters are inside the 100 trillion cells. This is called "intracellular" fluid. Fifteen of the forty liters comprises the fluid outside the cells; the extracellular fluid.

THE THREE FLUID COMPARTMENTS OF THE BODY

Fluid exists in three compartments, which are separated by a semipermeable membrane. In health there is a dynamic and proportionate equilibrium of fluid and electrolytes in the three compartments.

Fluid compartments	Amounts of fluid
Intracellular	25 to 27 liters (about two thirds of total body fluids, of which 2 liters is within the red blood cells)
Interstitial	10 liters (one fourth of total body fluids)
Intravascular (plasma)	3 to 5 liters (one twelfth of total body fluids)

Fluid within the three fluid compartments is either extracellular or intracellular fluid. This classification can be confusing. Intracellular fluid is that within *all* body cells; including the red and white blood cells and the tissue cells (muscle, nerve, connective, and epithelial). Interstitial fluid is all fluid outside of, or surrounding the tissue cells; hence, it is an extracellular fluid. Intravascular fluid consists of *both* intracellular and extracellular fluid. The fluid within the red blood cells is, of course, intracellular, while the plasma fluid is extracellular. (See Fig. 6.) The following outline shows the divisions of extracellular and intracellular fluid:

1. Extracellular fluid
   a. Interstitial fluid, which exists in the spaces between the tissue cells
   b. Plasma
   c. Cerebrospinal fluid
   d. Fluids of the gastrointestinal tract
   e. Fluids of the potential spaces
      (1) Potential pleural space
      (2) Peritoneal cavity

          (3) Pericardial cavity
          (4) All joint spaces
          (5) The bursae
      2. Intracellular fluid
        a. Red blood cells
        b. White blood cells
        c. All other body tissue cells

Water is freely movable between the three compartments, however, the solute concentration of electrolytes determines the volume within the three compartments. Sodium is the main solute of plasma and the interstitial compartment, hence, it determines the fluid volume in these areas.

The average blood volume of a normal-sized adult is almost exactly 5000 ml., of which 3000 ml. is plasma, and the remaining 2000 ml. of water is in the red blood cells. These values vary in different individuals; sex, weight, and other factors affect the blood volume.

ELECTROLYTES

All body fluids contain chemicals, or minerals called electrolytes. Electrolytes, by contributing to proper osmotic relationships, help to control the fluid volume of the body, help to maintain the acid-base balance, and provide proper ionic balance for normal tissue irritability and functioning. An electrolyte may be an acid, base, or salt that, in solution, has the power to conduct an electric current. Some electrolytes are more active, chemically, than others.

Electrolytes break up into ions; positively charged ions are called "cations," and negatively charged ions are called "anions."

Major cations in the body	Major anions in the body
Na^+ (sodium)	Cl^- (chlorine)
K^+ (potassium)	$(HCO3)^-$ (bicarbonate)
Ca^{++} (calcium)	$(HPO4^{--})$ (hydrogen phosphate)
Mg^{++} (magnesium)	$SO4^{--}$ (sulfate)

Each fluid compartment contains similar electrolytes, however, the concentration of electrolytes in each compartment varies markedly. Like the fluids of the body, the percentage of electrolytes remains remarkably constant in health, but can become markedly unbalanced in disease and shock.

The electrolyte concentration in interstitial fluid and plasma is very similar. However, the distinctive difference between them is the presence of approximately 7 gms./100 ml. of protein in the plasma.

The retention or elimination of water is a major means of maintaining a constant concentration of electrolytes. An excessive loss of body fluids (such as whole blood or plasma) may result in an electrolyte imbalance. The kidneys play an important role in the regulation of electrolyte concentrations, as they have the power to reabsorb sodium and chloride in the kidney tubules. This reabsorption process is influenced by several important hormones such as aldosterone and antidiuretic hormone (ADH). These will be discussed in proper context later.

The body cells and fluid normally maintain an osmotic pressure of about 0.9 per cent sodium chloride; this is an isotonic solution. An isotonic solution exerts the same osmotic pressure on one side of a semipermeable membrane as the solution on the other side of the membrane.

Sodium is the chief extracellular cation (existing in the plasma and interstitial compartment), and potassium is the chief intracellular cation. Potassium is roughly thirty-five times more concentrated in cells than it is in interstitial fluid or plasma. An increase, a decrease, or a displacement of sodium and/or potassium into another fluid compartment can prove very dangerous, if not fatal. We shall view this again in the discussion of acidosis.

The concentration of electrolytes in the interstitial fluid and in the plasma are very similar. The distinctive and important difference between them is the presence of approximately 7 gms./100 ml. of proteins in the plasma. It is this protein that creates the colloid osmotic pressure.

ACID-BASE BALANCE

For normal body-functioning, an acid-base ratio of 1:20 is requisite. The regulation of acid-base balance depends on three principal factors:

1. Buffer systems
2. Excretion of acid or alkali by the kidneys
3. Excretion of carbon dioxide by the lungs

Buffers convert strong acids and bases into weaker ones. Chief buffers of the blood are the following:

1. Carbonic acid (H_2CO_3) and its bicarbonate salt, $NaHCO_3$ (sodium bicarbonate)
2. Hemoglobin (Hgb), a weak acid

Carbonic acid is regulated by the respiratory system. All other electrolytes are under the control of the kidneys. There is a constant production of acid products from protein metabolism, lactic acid from muscle activity, and ketone acids from fats when carbohydrate levels are low.

Metabolism

PRINCIPLE 2: There is a direct relationship between metabolism and cellular requirements for oxygen, nutrients, water, electrolytes, and hormones.

a. Increased metabolism leads to an increased need of cells for oxygen, nutrients, water, electrolytes, and hormones.

b. Decreased metabolism leads to a decreased need of the cells for oxygen, nutrients, water, electrolytes, and hormones.

PRINCIPLE 3: In health, there is a relative and dynamic equilibrium between anabolism and catabolism.

Metabolism occurs at the cellular level and consists of two phases: (1) anabolism (building up), and (2) catabolism (breaking down). General metabolism includes the changes occurring in digested foods from the time of their absorption until their elimination in the excretions. In a more limited sense, metabolism refers to the sum total of chemical changes taking place within the cells. The rates of chemical reactions are, to a large extent, dependent on the amount of oxygen in the extracellular fluid. If oxygen is decreased, chemical reactions, and hence metabolism, decrease.

Metabolism is concerned with the manufacture of protoplasm in growth, maintenance and repair of tissue, and the provision of energy for cellular function.

Glucose is the major carbohydrate and, in the presence of oxygen, can be metabolized to carbon dioxide and water, with the release of energy. Enzymes are catalysts that speed chemical reactions and are responsible for the speed and efficiency with which energy is created within the cells. All digestive juices are catalysts.

PRINCIPLE 4. There is a direct relationship between cell activity and metabolic rate.

EFFECT OF AGE ON METABOLISM

The metabolic rate of the child is considerably higher than the adult's because the child needs more energy for the building of new tissue. With advancing age, the metabolic rate decreases.

EFFECT OF SEX ON METABOLISM

In health, the metabolic rate of the female is generally less than that of the male. During pregnancy and lactation however, the metabolic rate increases markedly.

EFFECT OF ILLNESS ON METABOLISM

Infections and other disease processes place greater demands on the body; hence, the metabolic rate is increased, as well as caloric requirements. The metabolic response to injury is a direct consequence of the neuroendocrine response.

Shock is characterized as a hypercatabolic response. The aims of treatment, in this instance, are to increase anabolism and to decrease catabolism. This has important implications for nursing care as we will see later on in the book.

EFFECT OF HORMONES ON METABOLISM

In general, increased hormonal activity leads to increased metabolism. Consider, for example, the increased metabolism of the hyperthyroid person, due to increased thyroxine. Hypothyroidism, on the other hand, causes a reduced metabolic rate. Severe depression of the thyroid gland leads to myxedema. Shock due to myxedema coma is associated with severe decrease of oxidative metabolism.

EFFECT OF TEMPERATURE ON METABOLISM

PRINCIPLE 5: The metabolic rate is related directly and proportionately to the body temperature.

a. As the body temperature increases, the metabolic rate increases.

b. As the body temperature decreases, the metabolic rate decreases.

When the body temperature increases, cardiac output and peripheral blood flow increase. Based on animal experiments, for each one degree Centigrade rise in body temperature, there is a 25 per cent increase in cardiac output.[2] An elevated body temperature also causes general peripheral vasodilatation, presumably in an effort to dissipate body heat. On the other hand, there is a decrease in cardiac output with hypothermia.

For each 1 degree Centigrade rise in body temperature, there is a 7 per cent increase in body metabolism. Fever accelerates all the body processes. Fever retards the growth of bacteria and decreases the potency of their toxins, as well as favoring phagocytosis and antibody formation.

EFFECTS OF SHOCK ON METABOLISM

All changes caused by shock can be regarded as metabolic abnormalities, since they result from changes in cell function and metabolism. Since shock represents a decreased supply of oxygen, nutrients, water, electrolytes, and hormones to the cells, cellular metabolism is decreased. For awhile, energy needs are supplied by anaerobic glycolysis. TO APPLY HEAT TO THE PATIENT IN SHOCK WOULD BE WRONG! Heat would increase his metabolic needs which, obviously, cannot be supplied by his body at this time. Since the five substances needed by the cells are delivered by the blood, which, in turn, is pumped by the heart, to apply heat to this patient would place an added burden on the heart. This could result in the demise of the cardiogenic shock patient.

EFFECT OF PREGNANCY ON METABOLISM

During pregnancy and lactation, the metabolic rate increases greatly. There are increases in cardiac output to values of 30 to 50 per cent above normal, until the end of the second trimester. Cardiac output declines in the last trimester. By the fortieth week of pregnancy, cardiac output returns to near normal. During delivery, cardiac output

---

[2] Max H. Weil, and Herbert Shubin, *Diagnosis & Treatment of Shock*, Baltimore: Williams & Wilkins Co., 1967, p. 52.

increases about 30 per cent, and immediately after delivery, cardiac output increases of 10 to 15 per cent have been observed.

EFFECTS OF PHYSICAL STRESS ON METABOLISM

Any stressor which is superimposed on a person in a poor nutritional state will add insult to injury on the body. The hormonal response to physical stress has an anabolic effect on other parts, with the total catabolism exceeding anabolism. For example, surgery, injury, fractures, and burns are accompanied by an increased loss of nitrogen, sulfur, phosphorus, potassium, and creatine, as well as essential nutrients. The glucose tolerance and serum cholesterol decrease, and there is a disturbance in electrolyte metabolism. The intense catabolism caused by severe stress is associated with loss of vitamin C, proteins, carbohydrates, and lipids.

REFERENCES

Baue, A. D. "Metabolic Abnormalities of Shock." *The Surgical Clinics of North America,* Philadelphia: W. B. Saunders Co., 1976, Vol. 56.

Beland, Irene L. *Clinical Nursing.* 2nd ed. New York: Macmillan Publishing Co., Inc. 1970.

Best and Taylor's. Physiological Basis of Medical Practice. 9th ed. John R. Brobeck (Ed.). Baltimore: Williams & Wilkins Co., 1973.

Chaffee, Ellen E., and Esther M. Greisheimer. *Basic Physiology and Anatomy,* 3rd ed. Philadelphia: J. B. Lippincott Co., 1974.

Hollenberg, N. K., and P. J. Cannon. "The Kidney in Congestive Heart Failure: Sodium Homeostasis, Renal Hemodynamics and Nephron Function." *Directions in Cardiovascular Medicine.* Hoechst-Roussel Pharmaceuticals, 1975.

Guyton, Arthur C. *Textbook of Medical Physiology,* 5th ed. Philadelphia: W. B. Saunders Co., 1976.

Selye, Hans. "On Just Being Sick." *Nutrition Today,* 5:2–10, 1970.

Sheldon, Alan, Frank Baker, and Curtis McLaughlin (Eds.). *Systems and Medical Care.* Cambridge, Mass.: The MIT Press, 1970.

Werko, L., H. Lagerhof, H. Bucht, and A. Holmgren. "Circulatory Changes in Pregnancy." (Abstract) *Acta Med. Scand.,* suppl. 239, 263, 1950.

CHAPTER 4

The Homeostasis of the Whole Body and Its Parts

PRINCIPLE 6: A state of health implies a dynamic equilibrium of the whole body—homeostasis.

PRINCIPLE 7: The health and life of an individual—cells, tissues, organs, and systems—are dependent on a sufficient supply of oxygen, nutrients, water, electrolytes, and hormones, and the removal of waste products.

Homeostasis

"Homeostasis" is a concept which describes the physiological mechanisms that protect and restore the normal. Maladaptive aspects of homeostasis include: (1) an excessive response, (2) a deficient response, or (3) an inappropriate response. When homeostatic mechanisms are elicited, the body engages in behavior that is directed toward reducing the tension.

Implicit in the normal healthy structure and functioning of the whole body is the health or homeostasis of all of its parts. This, in

31

turn, implies that there must be an adequate amount and delivery of oxygen, nutrients, water, electrolytes, and hormones to all body cells, and the removal of cellular waste products. If the four types of cells do not receive the five substances necessary for their health and activity, then neither do the tissues, organs, body systems, and total organism.

Predicated in this is the homeostasis of respiration, circulation, nutrition, fluid and electrolyte, and nervous and hormonal control mechanisms. Failure of any one part of any of these would represent an imbalance, or maladaptive homeostatic state.

The Homeostasis of Respiration: Internal and External

PRINCIPLE 8:   Oxygen is necessary to sustain life.

Survival of an organism is dependent upon a functioning respiratory system with an adequate exchange of oxygen and carbon dioxide. Many tissues, including the myocardium, peripheral blood vessels, and central nervous system are exquisitely sensitive to short periods of extreme lack of oxygen. An increased accumulation of high levels of carbon dioxide is rapidly destructive of myocardial action and peripheral vascular tone.

External respiration is the exchange of oxygen and carbon dioxide between the lungs and the atmosphere. Internal respiration is the exchange of oxygen and carbon dioxide at the cell level.

PRINCIPLE 9:   The amount of gas that can diffuse across a membrane is proprotionate to the quantity and partial pressure of the gas and the circumference of the surface area of the membrane with which the gas is in direct contact.

By the process of diffusion, oxygen enters the blood stream and ultimately crosses the cell membrane into the cell. Let us see how this is accomplished. At the completion of inspiration, oxygen is more highly concentrated in the alveoli of the lungs than it is in the venous blood of the pulmonary capillary blood stream. Since the wall of the alveolus is a permeable membrane, the oxygen within the alveolus, assisted by a partial pressure of gases, diffuses across the alveolar membrane into the pulmonary capillary blood stream. At the same time, carbon dioxide (the chief cellular waste product), which is more concentrated in the pulmonary capillary blood stream than it is in the alveolus,

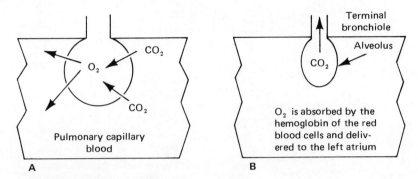

Figure 5. *Normal respiratory exchange of gases.*
A. Normal inspiration. Normal diffusion of oxygen and carbon dioxide.
B. Normal expiration. Note the elastic recoil of the alveolus which forces carbon dioxide out of the respiratory passages.

diffuses into the alveolus from whence it is exhaled from the respiratory tract. The diffusion of these two gases into and out of the pulmonary capillary blood stream is referred to as external respiration.

PRINCIPLE 10: The amount of oxygen that can be transported by the red blood cells is directly proportionate to the number of red blood cells and the amount of hemoglobin within the red cells.

Having diffused into the blood steam, the oxygen is picked up and carried by the hemoglobin which is a part of the red blood cells. The determination of the hemoglobin is often of greater importance than the red blood cell count itself. A person's red cell count might be normal, yet each red cell might contain less than the normal amount of hemoglobin. If 100 ml. of blood contains 7 or 8 gm. of hemoglobin, instead of the normal amount of 15 gm., the hemoglobin is only 50 per cent of normal. This person would be anemic and handicapped by a defective oxygen transport, even though his red cell count might be normal. Thus, an insufficient amount of hemoglobin implies a deficient supply of oxygen to the body cells.

As the blood reaches the capillaries of the body tissues, the oxygen diffuses across the capillary membrane into the interstitial compartment. From there, it diffuses across the cell membrane. At the same time, carbon dioxide leaves the cell, enters the interstitial compartment, and enters the capillary blood stream at the venous end. While oxygen is carried by the iron (heme) of the hemoglobin, the carbon

33

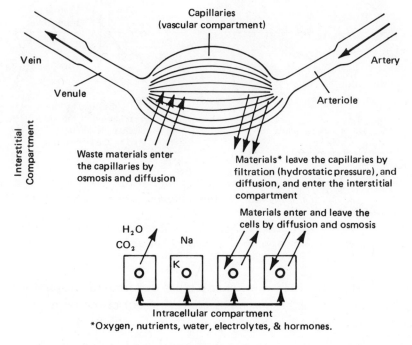

Figure 6. *Exchange of materials between fluid compartments.*

dioxide is carried by the protein portion (globin). Carbon dioxide is one of the chief endproducts of chemical changes occurring in the cells; hence, it must be eliminated continuously. Remember, normal respiration performs two important functions: (1) to supply oxygen to the cells, and (2) to remove carbon dioxide from the body.

Considered separately (and in order) to maintain an adequate supply of oxygen to all body cells, the following are requisite to maintain the homeostasis of respiration.

THE HOMEOSTASIS OF RESPIRATION: REQUISITES

1. An adequate supply of oxygen in the air
2. Stimulation of respiration (in the blood of the medulla oblongata)*

* The medulla oblongata contains many of the vital centers which are essential to life: (a) the respiratory center, to change the rate and depth of breathing, (b) the cardiac center to accelerate or slow the heart rate, (c) the vasomotor center to constrict or dilate the blood vessels, and (d) reflex centers: coughing, sneezing, vomiting, and swallowing.

    a. By decreased oxygen in the blood, *or*

    b. Increased carbon dioxide, *or*

    c. Increased hydrogen ions

3. An open airway through which the oxygen can pass to the alveoli

    a. Open nares, unobstructed

    b. Pharynx

    c. Larynx

    d. Trachea

    e. Main bronchi

    f. Bronchial tubes

    g. Bronchioles

4. Alveoli of

    a. Sufficient number

    b. Elasticity

    c. Thin membranes

    d. Surfactant in the alveoli (a lack of which leads to collapsed alveoli, atelectasis, and pneumonia).

5. Expanded lungs: negative pressure between the visceral and parietal pleurae of the lungs, to maintain them in an expanded and symetrically rhythmic state, intact rib cage, and internal and external intercostal muscles to allow for chest expansion.

6. Intact diaphragm (innervated by intact phrenic nerves) with the ability to expand and contract; to pull the oxygen into the lungs, and to relax & push the carbon dioxide from the lungs.

7. An adequate pulmonary blood supply with a sufficient quantity and quality of red blood cells.

8. A healthy heart to pump the oxygenated blood to all parts of the body.

9. Cells that can utilize the oxygen.

Anything that interferes with, or disrupts any one or more of the listed chain of events, will lead to decreased oxygen supply to the cells, tissues, organs, systems, and whole organism. Hence, signs and symptoms of oxygen deficiency will become manifest.

As a result, it is not difficult to understand how the following can cause decreased oxygenation to the cells:

Hemorrhage

Anemia

Heart failure
Pneumothorax
Atelectasis
Pulmonary emphysema
Diaphragmatic hernia
Myasthenia gravis
Obstruction of any part of the airway
And so on

The difficulty lies in assessing the underlying *cause* of the decreased oxygenation to the cells. Any failure in the respiratory process must be dealt with specifically. For example, to correct the oxygen deficiency of a patient with hemorrhage, the implied treatment is to replace the blood volume in order to supply sufficient red blood cells and hemoglobin to *carry* the oxygen. The hypoxic person might have a sufficient blood supply, but may have increased mucous in his bronchi. Suctioning and/or coughing would be in order for this person, so as to increase the diameter of the tube through which oxygen can again pass.

The person in anaphylactic shock may be hypoxic due to severe bronchiolar constriction. Giving blood would not help this person, nor suctioning. What he needs is a bronchodilator drug, such as adrenalin, to overcome the bronchiolar constriction. Although the administration of oxygen might be of some help to the person with a decreased blood volume or anemia, oxygen would be of little help to the person in anaphylactic shock because its passage through the bronchiolar tube system would be obstructed.

Succinctly, the *cause* should determine the nursing care and treatment. This is the meaning of scientific nursing care. This is the basis of a *meaningful* nursing assessment, or, if you prefer, nursing diagnosis.

The Homeostasis of the Circulation of the Blood

PRINCIPLE 11: Adequate circulation of blood to all body parts is dependent upon a proportionate equilibrium between the blood volume, the strength of cardiac contractions, and the size of the lumina of the blood vessels.

The delivery of the five substances to the four types of cells, and the removal of cell wastes are the major functions of the circulatory system.

Circulatory homeostasis implies that there is a dynamic equilibrium and interrelationship between the blood volume, cardiac pump action, and the size of the diameter of the blood vessels. Simply, shock threatens from the weakness or failure of any one of these three mechanisms. It is interesting to note that, in line with the interdependence implicit in the systems theory, with the failure of any one of the three mechanisms, the other two will compensate for the deficiency for awhile, in order to sustain life.

HOMEOSTASIS OF CIRCULATION: REQUISITES

Normal circulation of blood throughout the body implies the following requisites:

1. Blood of sufficient quantity and quality
   a. Sufficient red blood cells
   b. Sufficient hemoglobin in the red blood cells
   c. Sufficient plasma
2. A healthy heart to pump the blood, under pressure, through
3. An intact and patent circulatory circuit
   a. Arteries and arterioles
      (1) Of the proper diameter (resistance)
      (2) Elasticity of the vessels
   b. Intact and patent capillaries with the proper degree of
      (1) Hydrostatic filtration pressure within them
      (2) Permeability
   c. Patent and intact venules and veins of the proper diameter
4. Patent lymphatics to convey excess small proteins and water to the venous system
5. A healthy venous pump to propel the venous blood to the right atrium
   (1) Valves in the veins to prevent backflow
   (2) Skeletal muscles ⎫ to milk the blood back
   (3) Diaphragm ⎭ to the right atrium
6. A healthy respiratory system for the diffusion of carbon dioxide and oxygen from and into the blood, respectively.

Failure of any one or more of the listed requisites will ultimately result in a decreased amount of the five substances to the four types of cells. Hence, decreased cellular energy will result and will be manifest by signs and symptoms at the cell, tissue, organ, and systems levels. In turn, these signs and symptoms will be reflected by the whole organism.

Let us consider the salient features of each of these requisites.

Blood of sufficient quantity and quality

In the adult, the normal blood volume is about four to five liters, of which red blood cells constitute 45 per cent of the volume, and plasma constitutes 55 per cent. In health, the blood volume remains remarkably constant. The two major factors in its regulation are

1. The colloid osmotic pressure (C.O.P.) of the plasma proteins in the vascular compartment, and
2. The hydrostatic pressure of the blood within the capillaries.

Blood carries the five substances to the cells, it carries away the waste products, it fights infection, and it plays a vital role in the adjustment of the temperature, acid-base balance, and fluid balance.

Hemoglobin combines with oxygen to form oxyhemoglobin, which gives the bright scarlet color to oxygenated blood. When the hemoglobin gives up its oxygen in the capillaries, the blood becomes darker. This is referred to as "reduced" hemoglobin. In women the hemoglobin content of the blood is 14 gm., and in men it averages about 16 gm. In hemorrhage and anemia the hemoglobin is lower than normal, hence the oxygen-carrying power is decreased. According to Secor, "analysis of arterial blood reflects ventilation efficiency, the ability of hemoglobin to carry oxygen and carbon dioxide, the rate of cellular metabolism, and the state of the buffer system."[1]

The hematocrit of the blood is the percentage that is red blood cells. For example, a hematocrit of 40 means that 40 percent of the blood volume is red blood cells; the remainder is plasma. The normal hematocrit in woman is 38, and in man it is 42.

There is a direct relationship between the hematocrit and the viscosity of the blood; as the hematocrit increases, the viscosity increases. Thick, highly viscous blood with its clumped cells is referred to as sludged blood. This is abnormal, and could prove dangerous in clot formation. Daily hematocrits will aid in determining continued loss of blood from trauma areas, stress ulcers, and so on.

---

[1] Jane Secor, *Patient Care in Respiratory Problems*, Saunders Monograph in Clinical Nursing I. Philadelphia: W. B. Saunders Co., 1969, p. 85.

PRINCIPLE 12:   Anything that causes an increase in the number of red blood cells, or that decreases the plasma volume will lead to an increase in the viscosity of the blood.

PRINCIPLE 13:   There is an inverse relationship between the viscosity of the blood and the velocity of blood flow.

  a. An increased viscosity leads to a decreased velocity.

  b. A decreased viscosity leads to an increased velocity.

The plasma is composed of approximately 92 per cent water, and 6 to 8 per cent proteins (albumin-globulin), plus various electrolytes; the predominant ones being sodium and chloride. The plasma electrolytes regulate fluid balance, and, partly because of their buffering action, they also help to regulate the acid-base balance.

Of the plasma proteins, albumin plays a very important osmotic role, as it is mostly responsible for the colloid osmotic pressure (oncotic pressure) of the plasma; hence, it helps to regulate the volume of plasma within the capillaries by pulling fluid from the interstitial compartment into the capillaries. The control of the blood volume depends upon intake and output of water and electrolytes, and on the movement of fluid among the vascular, interstitial, and intracellular compartments. Protein, especially the albumin of the plasma, is of prime importance in determining the distribution of fluid among the three fluid compartments. The adrenal glands play a major role in the control of the volume of plasma and protein, and therefore in the homeostatic regulation of the blood volume.

Following hemorrhage, when whole blood is not available, an albumin solution may be ordered intravenously to increase the blood volume by pulling fluid, osmotically, into the vascular compartment from the interstitial compartment. In the burned patient who has lost vast quantities of fluid and plasma into the interstitial compartment, as a result of damaged capillaries (hence increased capillary permeability), plasma is often given to replace and to remobilize the fluid back into the vascular compartment.

A HEALTHY HEART TO PUMP THE BLOOD, UNDER PRESSURE, THROUGH AN INTACT CIRCULATORY CIRCUIT

PRINCIPLE 14:   The proper functioning of all body tissues is dependent on a sufficient quality and volume of blood flowing under sufficient pressure.

PRINCIPLE 15: An adequate cardiac output is basic to the health and proper functioning of all body tissues.

PRINCIPLE 16: The heart can eject into the arterial circuit only that amount of blood it receives from the venous circuit.

PRINCIPLE 17: A constant supply of blood and the removal of wastes from the myocardium are basic for adequate myocardial contractions.

The heart

Because of the valves between the left atrium and left ventricle; left ventricle and aorta; right atrium and right ventricle; right ventricle and pulmonary artery, blood cannot regurgitate.

Since the heart pump, itself, is an organ composed of tissue and cells, it needs fresh supplies of blood to deliver nutrients and oxygen to it, and to remove its waste products. The blood vessels through which the heart receives its fresh supply of blood are the right and left coronary arteries which arise from the aortic sinus. The coronary veins remove the waste products from the cardiac tissue and empty them into the right atrium.

The myocardium provides the pumping power that propels the blood, on systole, from the right and left ventricles. When the myocardium relaxes in the diastolic phase, it receives a fresh supply of blood from the coronary arteries. In order to function effectively as a pump, the myocardium requires a sufficient blood supply. When the supply of fresh blood does not meet the demands of the myocardium, a relative degree of myocardial failure ensues.

The law of the heart is frequently referred to as Starling's Law. Fundamentally, Starling's Law states that the greater the heart is filled during diastole, the greater will be the force of cardiac contraction, and, as a consequence, the greater also will be the amount of blood pumped out of the heart.

Myocardial contractility is also influenced by sympathetic activity, aortic pressure, heart rate, and coronary blood flow. Roughly, at rest, healthy cardiac output is distributed thusly: 25 per cent to the kidneys, 15 per cent to the brain, 10 per cent to the coronary artery, 15 per cent to the liver, 10 per cent to the skin, 15 per cent to muscles, and 10 per cent to other viscera. During exercise, the amount of blood flow to the muscles increases very much, as it does to the skin in warm or hot environments.[2]

[2] Alan C. Burton, *Physiology and Biophysics of the Circulation,* Chicago: Year Book Medical Publishers, 1965, p. 15.

From the arteries the blood flows through the arterioles which end at the capillaries. At the capillaries oxygen, nutrients, water, electrolytes, and hormones pass from the blood stream by crossing the capillary membrane, enter the interstitial compartment, and diffuse into the cell. At the venous end of the capillary bed, excess fluid passes through the capillary membrane by the process of osmosis, and gaseous wastes diffuse into the capillary. These are conveyed through the veins to the right atrium of the heart. From the right atrium the deoxygenated venous blood passes into the right ventricle, from which it is pumped through the pulmonary artery to the lungs. In the pulmonary capillary blood stream, the main waste product (carbon dioxide) diffuses from the blood stream into the alveoli and is exhaled. After picking up oxygen from the pulmonary alveoli, the fresh blood then flows via the four pulmonary veins to the left atrium and then to the left ventricle. This cycle repeats until death.

The pulse

When the left ventricle contracts, blood is forced along through the arterial vessels, producing a wave which is felt in the distended blood vessels. The crest of the wave corresponds with the contraction, or systole, of the heart. Both upward and downward curves constitute the pulse and represent one complete heart beat—contraction and relaxation, or systole and diastole. The pulse beat consists of two phases; the ebb and the crest. It is the crest which we feel when checking the pulse. When counting the pulse, one should start with the count of zero, then count 1, 2, 3, and so on for subsequent beats. Failure to do so will give an inaccurate count, since the first beat we feel constitutes only half of the pulse cycle.[3]

An increase in body temperature causes an increase in the heart rate of approximately twenty beats per degree Centigrade above normal in the adult. The pulse rate also increases with anger and fear.

The pulse is a reflection of the heart beat. When one rests, the tissues require less blood; therefore, the heart beats slower and is reflected in the slow beat of the pulse. On the other hand, when one exercises, more blood is needed by the tissues, and the demands for blood are met by a rapid heart beat which is reflected in a rapid pulse beat. In this way, the heart compensates for the burdens placed on the body by increased metabolism.

[3] Ibid, p. 158.

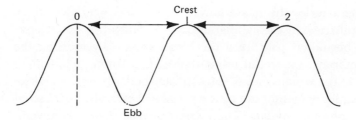

Figure 7. *The pulse (ebb and crest).*

PRINCIPLE 18:   There is a direct relationship between metabolic rate and cardiac rate.
    a. Increased metabolism increases the heart rate.
    b. Decreased metabolism decreases the heart rate.

Anything that increases body metabolism will increase the cardiac rate, and this is inclusive of physical and mental stress. In nature, parts develop in proportion to the stresses and strains placed upon them. To use one of many possible examples, the heart of an athelete enlarges (hypertrophies) in order to meet increasing cellular requirements.

BLOOD PRESSURE

PRINCIPLE 19:   The rate at which blood will flow through a blood vessel is determined by the pressure difference at each end of the vessel, the resistance to blood flow, and the viscosity of the blood.

The blood flows through the arterial blood vessels under pressure. Without pressure being exerted, the blood could not possibly reach the many capillary beds, and, if the reader recalls, in the absence of hydrostatic pressure at the arterial end of the capillary bed, there would be very little passage of substances from the vascular compartment into the interstitial compartment.

Definition of blood pressure

Blood pressure is the lateral pressure exerted by the blood on the walls of the vessels. The term "blood pressure" usually refers to the pressure of blood on the walls of the artery.

The traditional method of checking the arterial blood pressure is with a sphygmomanometer. It is anticipated, however, that in the near future intra-arterial methods of monitoring the blood pressure will be used routinely in the management of high risk patients in protracted shock. Measurements of intra-arterial pressure provide a far greater accuracy than measurements with a sphygmomanometer. In comparison with intra-arterial pressure, the cuff pressure is between 5 and 20 mm. Hg. lower in patients with clinical features of shock.

As the heart contracts, blood is forced out into the aorta and thus to the large arterial branches. The force of the blood exerted against the walls of the arteries represents the systolic blood pressure. The diastolic pressure represents the resting phase of the heart between beats, and is also a measure of peripheral resistance. Peripheral resistance, in turn, depends mainly on the tone of the arterioles. The diastolic pressure is normally 35 to 50 mm. Hg. lower than the systolic pressure.

Consider, for example, a soft plastic garden hose connected to a water faucet—the hose representing an artery, and the faucet representing the left ventricle. Turn on the faucet full-force and see, or feel, how the water, surging through the hose, exerts pressure on the inner wall of the hose. This is analagous to the systolic pressure, the contracting, or working period of the heart.

Now, turn off the faucet and see how the hose becomes limp. This represents the diastolic pressure, the resting period of the heart when the pressure of the blood against the arterial walls is decreased. Observe the end of the hose as you turn the faucet on and off, on and off, on and off. Note how the water is ejected forcefully each time you turn on the faucet, the result of systole. Note how the water ceases to come out of the end of the hose when you turn the faucet off, the result of diastole. Fluids flow from points of greater pressure to points of lesser pressure. Because the pressure at the open end of the hose is less than the pressure forcing the water through the hose, the water comes out of the open end. If a plug, however, were inserted at the end of the hose so the water could not come out, the pressure exerted against the inner wall of the hose would increase. Now, compare the faucet, the water, and the hose to the heart, the blood, and the arteries, and you will have a working example of the blood pressure.

Needless to say, the blood, in order to reach all parts of the body via the arterial vessels, needs to be moved through the blood vessels under pressure by the systolic efforts of the heart. A decrease in systole would result in a decreased supply of blood to body parts, which, in turn, implies a relative degree of hypoxia and decreased nutrition of body cells, along with a decreased removal of cellular waste products,

43

of which carbon dioxide is the dominant waste product, or metabolite. The blood pressure, then, must be of sufficient amplitude to force blood to all parts of the body.

The blood pressure is not determined by the systolic force of the heart, alone. The blood pressure is the result of five factors:

1. The force of the heart beat
2. The blood volume
3. The elasticity of the blood vessels
4. The size of the diameter of the lumen of blood vessels
5. The viscosity of the blood.

A weak heart beat results in the ejection of less blood from the heart, thus creating a lower blood pressure. Or, if blood is forced through a narrow, inelastic arterial system, such as occurs in arteriosclerosis, the blood pressure increases because the lumen of the vessel is smaller, and the walls are more rigid (less elastic). Because of the increased resistance to blood flow, the blood flows under increased pressure.

If blood is forced through dilated arteries (which implies an increased size of the diameter of the lumina of the vessels), there will be less resistance to the flow of blood, and the blood pressure will decrease. If a decreased volume of blood is forced through the arteries, the blood pressure would decrease, because the resistance of the blood against the walls of the vessels is decreased. On the other hand, an increased volume of blood would result in an increase in blood pressure.

"Viscosity" of the blood refers to its thinness or thickness. In the example of the faucet, water, and hose, one has to substitute oil for the water to understand the implications of viscosity. Oil, being more viscous (thicker) than water, would exert a greater pressure against the wall of the hose. The viscosity of the blood is dependent almost entirely on the concentration of red blood cells. In health, blood is three times as viscous as water. The viscosity of the blood varies with different conditions. At the onset of hemorrhage, the blood becomes more viscous, because red blood cells in excess are produced by the bone marrow and are squeezed from the liver, spleen, and venous reservoir into the circulatory stream in an effort to make up for those that have been lost. Although increased viscosity of the blood is accompanied by certain dangers, it also helps to increase the vascular resistance to blood flow, thus raising the blood pressure.

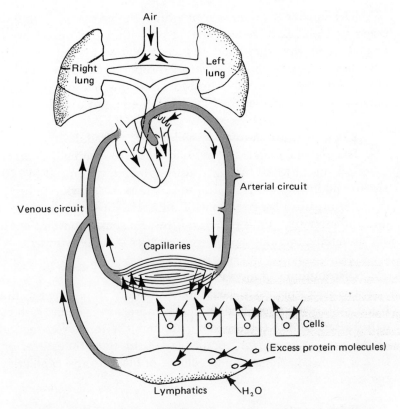

Figure 8. *The lungs, heart, and circulatory circuit. The heart in diastole— arterial blood from the lungs is delivered to the left atrium via the four pulmonary veins. The left atrium empties into the left ventricle. The venae cavae empty venous blood into the right atrium. The right atrium empties venous blood into the right ventricle.*

RHEOLOGY (The Flow of Blood)

Blood does not flow through the blood vessels as an exact cylinder; it flows in layers. The layer of blood next to the vessel wall moves more slowly, if at all. The next layer moves more rapidly, sliding over the outermost layer. The flow of blood is greatest in the center, or axis, of the vessels. This is referred to as *axial flow.* Therefore, if the viscosity of the blood is increased, sludging of the blood next to the vessel wall can readily occur. Sludging, in turn, can predispose to thrombi formation.

The smaller the diameter of a tube, the greater will be the resistance to blood flow; hence, the blood within the tube flows faster. Dilatation, on the other hand, reduces the flow of blood. Or, we might say that resistance to flow is inversely proportional to the fourth power of the diameter of the tube. Resistance to flow is also directly proportional to the viscosity of the blood and the length of the blood vessel.

Blood pressure in infancy, childhood, and adult life

During childhood, the systolic pressure gradually increases. It ranges from 75 to 90 mm. Hg. during infancy, from 90 to 110 mm. Hg. in childhood, and from 100 to 120 mm. Hg. during puberty. The diastolic pressure ranges about 50 mm. Hg. in the first few years of life, and after that, until puberty, it remains fairly constant at 60 mm. Hg. In adults, the blood pressure increases steadily with age.

Distribution of blood volume

Under normal conditions, approximately 70 per cent of the total blood volume is contained in the low-pressure venous system, and only 15 per cent in the arteries. Although the total cross-section area of the capillaries and/or venules is 700 to 1000 times greater than that of the aorta the maximal volume of blood in the capillaries is 12 per cent of the total volume.

Pulse pressure

The difference between the systolic and diastolic blood pressures is called the pulse pressure. The relation between the pulse pressure and the stroke volume of the heart gives a most useful index of changes in cardiac output. Cardiac output = stroke volume × heart rate. At rest, a blood pressure of 120/80, and a heart rate of 70 would yield 40 pulse pressure × 70 beats per minute = 2800 ml. of blood ejected from the heart per minute. In heavy exercise, if the blood pressure is 180/90, and the heart rate is 100 per minute, then pulse pressure × heart rate is 90 × 100 = 9000 ml.

$$\text{Pulse pressure} = \frac{\text{Stroke volume}}{\text{Arterial distensibility}}$$

Stroke volume = pulse pressure × arterial distensibility.

There is an inverse relationship between the pulse pressure and the elasticity and distensibility of the aorta and arteries. Therefore, increased elasticity of the aorta and arteries leads to a decreased (narrow) pulse pressure. Conversely, decreased elasticity of the aorta and arteries leads to an increased (widened) pulse pressure.

The normal pulse pressure is 40 mm. Hg. For example, a blood pressure of 120/80 would yield a pulse pressure of 40. In early stages of shock, the systolic pressure usually falls before the diastolic does. Therefore, the pulse pressure will be narrow. For example, a blood pressure of 100/76 yields a pulse pressure of 24. As shock progresses, the diastolic pressure will decrease further.

The pulse pressure is the result of two major factors: (1) the amount of blood that is ejected from the left ventricle during systole (the stroke volume), and (2) the distensibility of the arteries, i.e., how much the arteries can stretch when blood is forced out of the left ventricle of the heart. When the arterial resistance is decreased (vasodilatation), this allows a rapid flow of blood from the arteries to the veins. This increases venous return of blood to the right atrium which, in turn, results in an increased stroke volume and an increase in pulse pressure.

An increase in heart rate leads to a decrease in the heart's stroke volume, because of the shortened diastolic filling time of the heart. The pulse pressure, in this instance, decreases accordingly.

MEAN ARTERIAL PRESSURE (M.A.P.)

The mean arterial pressure determines the average rate at which blood will flow through the systemic vessels; hence, it reflects the tissue blood flow. If the mean arterial pressure falls too low, serious tissue damage results because of inadequate tissue perfusion.

The average pressure during one cardiac cycle is called the mean arterial pressure (M.A.P.). If the length of systole and diastole were equal, they could be averaged to obtain a close approximation of the mean arterial pressure. Systole, however, is usually of shorter duration than diastole. Therefore, the M.A.P. can be estimated as two thirds of the diastolic pressure plus one third of the systolic pressure, allowing for the longer period of diastole. Hence, the formula:

$$\text{M.A.P.} = \frac{1 \text{ systolic} + 2 \text{ diastolic}}{3}$$

With a blood pressure of 120/80, the M.A.P. would be approximately

$$93 \text{ mm. Hg.} \quad \frac{120 + 80 + 80}{3} = \frac{280}{3} = 93.3 \text{ mm Hg.}$$

The normal rate of urine formation by the kidneys is about 1 ml. per minute, or 60 ml. per hour. The production of urine by the kidneys requires a mean arterial pressure of around 70 mm. Hg. If the M.A.P. is lower than 70 mm. Hg, glomerular filtration rate (GFR) is markedly reduced and oliguria or anuria will result. If the low M.A.P. is prolonged, renal tubular necrosis will follow.

The production of urine is a good indication that the visceral organs are being perfused with blood.

THE BLOOD VESSELS

There are three principal classes of blood vessels, each of which is characterized by both structural and functional differences:

1. Arteries and arterioles. A high-pressure distributing system carrying oxygenated blood from the left side of the heart to all regions of the body. These are referred to as *resistance* vessels.
2. Capillaries. A low-pressure system of very minute vessels with extremely thin walls through which substances are exchanged between the vascular and interstitial compartments.
3. Veins and venules. A low-pressure collecting system which returns the deoxygenated blood to the right side of the heart. These are referred to as the *capacitance* vessels.

The blood flows from the left ventricle to the aorta, to large arteries, to smaller arteries, to arterioles and metarterioles, to capillaries, where changes of supplies and wastes take place, to venules, to small veins, to larger veins, to the venae cavae, to the right atrium. In some terminal regions of the body, however, the blood flows in an alternative route, from terminal arterioles to distal veins, thus bypassing the capillaries. This circulatory pattern is referred to as *arterio-venous shunt.* Arteriovenous shunts are relatively numerous in the skin—covering the fingers, toes, nose, lips, and ears. The shunts play a role in the regulation of the temperature of these tissues which are intimately exposed to variations in environmental temperature.

Arteries and arterioles

The aorta, arising from the left ventricle, is the largest artery and is about one inch in diameter. Arteries of various sizes branch off the aorta, and, in turn, divide and subdivide into smaller and smaller arteries called arterioles and metarterioles. The arterioles extend to all regions of the body. Metarterioles are tiny arterioles immediately preceding the capillaries.

Arterial layers. Arteries are composed of three circular layers. 1. Inner layer. It is composed of smooth endothelial cells and a band of elastic tissue. 2. Middle layer. It consists mainly of smooth involuntary muscle arranged in a circular fashion, and elastic tissue. The elastic tissue predominates in the larger arteries, while the smooth muscle predominates in the small arteries. The muscle fibers comprising the walls of the middle layer of arteries are arranged in a circular fashion and are involuntary, meaning that they cannot be controlled by will. There are two exceptions to this; the brain and the heart have a very carefully autoregulated flow which is independent of the automatic sympathetic nervous system. Thus, when the sympathetic vasomotor nerves cause constriction of the middle layer of the blood vessels, the peripheral arteriolar blood flow is diverted to the brain and heart to meet their metabolic needs. This is one of the many compensatory mechanisms occurring in shock. What a beautiful example of interdependence!

The role of the vasomotor nerves

Vaso refers to blood vessel, and *motor* refers to action upon. The middle layer of the arterioles is composed of a highly developed muscle layer which is capable of varying the diameter of the arteriolar lumen. For example, the contraction of the smooth muscle layer causes the diameter of the lumen to become smaller; this is called *vasoconstriction.* The greater the constriction, the greater is the arteriolar resistance and diastolic blood pressure. On the other hand, relaxation of the muscle layer causes the lumen to become larger; this is called *vasodilatation.* The greater the dilatation, the lower is the arteriolar resistance and diastolic blood pressure.

The vasomotor nerves consist of two types: the vasoexcitors which cause vasoconstriction, and the vasoinhibitors which cause vasodilatation. The vasomotor center located in the medulla oblongata of the brain is highly sensitive to the gaseous composition of the blood flowing through its vessels. A high carbon dioxide tension or a low oxygen tension causes an increase in vasoconstrictor tone with a resulting increase in blood pressure. In acute conditions such as shock, vasoconstriction preserves blood flow in certain vital regions at the expense of less vital parts.

The net effect of sympathetic vasomotor stimulation of the veins is:

1. Venous constriction, hence an initial decreased venous capacitance,
2. Increased amounts of venous blood empty into the right atrium,
3. Increased cardiac output which leads to an increased systolic blood pressure.

Emotions and vasomotor activity. We know that emotional stimuli elicit vasomotor activity. Increasing levels of excitement are associated with increasing degrees of vasoconstriction. States of depression often cause the opposite effect, i.e., vasodilatation.

Effects of the size of the diameter of blood vessels on blood flow. The size of the diameter of a blood vessel affects the flow of the blood in proportion to the fourth power of the diameter of the vessel. Very slight changes in the diameter will cause a tremendous change in flow. (See Fig. 9.) Changes in the length of a vessel, the viscosity of the blood, or pressure affect blood flow to a far lesser extent.

Blood flow = velocity × area.

$$\text{Velocity} = \frac{\text{blood flow}}{\text{diameter}}$$

Figure 9. *Resistance to blood flow is inversely proportional to the fourth power of a vessel's diameter.*

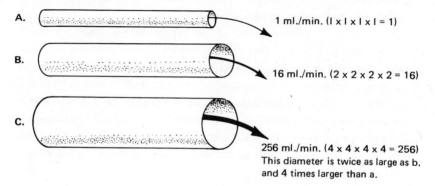

A. 1 ml./min. (l x l x l x l = 1)

B. 16 ml./min. (2 x 2 x 2 x 2 = 16)

C. 256 ml./min. (4 x 4 x 4 x 4 = 256)
This diameter is twice as large as b. and 4 times larger than a.

Resistance to blood flow is inversely proportional to the fourth power of a vessel's diameter. It can be seen in Fig. 9 that blood flow and blood pressure are markedly affected by relatively small changes in the size of a vessel's diameter.

The capillaries

The distal parts of the arterial tree are made up of arterioles which lead into a system of minute vessels called capillaries. Capillaries connect the arterial and venous systems. Despite the very small diameter of their luminae, the blood flows more slowly through the capillaries than it does through the larger arteries and veins because the sum total of the capillary diameters is greater than the diameter of any artery or vein leading to and from them, respectively.

There is a steady flow of blood into the capillaries. The elastic arteries accomodate extra blood forced into them during systole, and recoil on diastole, thus forcing blood toward the capillaries. Blood flow through the capillaries is nonpulsatile.

Velocity of blood flow

The velocity of blood flow varies inversely with the cross-sectional area; the larger the diameter of a vessel, the slower the flow of blood; and the smaller the diameter, the faster the flow. The blood pressure within the latter would be greater. Approximate illustrative values for velocity and relative values for cross-sectional areas in the various divisions of the circulatory system are

Division	Relative area of Cross Section	Blood velocity
Arterial (aorta)	1	22 cm per second
Venous (venae cavae)	2	11 cm per second
Capillaries	600–800	0.1 to 0.05 cm per second

All gaseous and fluid exchanges between the blood and the interstitial compartment take place across the capillary membrane. The arteries and veins are impervious. As can be seen in Fig. 6, materials leave and enter the blood stream at the capillary level. At no other place in the circulatory circuit can this occur. The marked slowing of the blood flow within the capillaries allows time for the exchange to occur. The capillaries, then, are the only functional units, so far as

51

appreciable exchange of materials between the blood and tissues is concerned, and the entire circulatory circuit—the heart, arteries, arterioles, venules, and veins, with all their controlling mechanisms—functions to serve the capillaries.

The capillary wall (membrane). The state of the capillary wall, or membrane, with respect to permeability is of utmost importance in maintaining the nutrition of the tissues and in maintaining the normal distribution of fluids in and out of the vascular compartment. The capillary membrane is porous and extremely thin, and is composed of a single layer of endothelial cells. The membrane is bound together by a cementlike substance; an alteration in the cement substance changes the permeability of the capillary. The size of the pores of its semipermeable membrane varies from small to large, the larger pores permitting larger molecules to pass through. Many conditions can affect the permeability of capillary membranes: trauma (the reader is familiar with the bruise caused by trauma), lack of vitamin C, hypoxia, heat, decreased calcium salts, leukotaxin, and histamine are a few that cause increased capillary permeability. On the other hand, capillary permeability can be decreased by the following: cooling to a temperature that does not cause tissue injury, calcium salts, and adrenal corticoids.

Factors determining the movement of substances through capillaries

The four primary factors that determine whether fluid will move out of the vascular compartment into the interstitial compartment, or vice versa, are:

1. The *capillary pressure* (hydrostatic pressure), which tends to move fluid outward through the capillary membrane into the interstitial compartment.
2. The *interstitial fluid pressure* which tends to move fluid through the capillary membrane into the vascular compartment.
3. The *plasma colloid osmotic pressure* (C.O.P.) which causes osmosis of fluid into the vascular compartment from the interstitial compartment.
4. The *interstitial fluid colloid osmotic pressure* which tends to cause osmosis of fluid from the vascular to the interstitial com-

partment, as well as retaining fluid in the interstitial compartment.

Capillary pressure. When the capillary hydrostatic pressure falls too low, large amounts of fluid from the interstitial compartment begin to pass into the vascular compartment, thereby rapidly increasing the blood volume until the capillary pressure returns to its normal level. Thus it can be seen how the body protects itself when a loss of blood volume, and/or a decreased blood pressure threaten it.

If the capillary pressure rises too high, excessive fluid will leak out of the vascular compartment, thereby decreasing the circulating blood volume, and again returning the capillary pressure to its equilibrium value.

Increased capillary pressure can result from any condition that causes either venous obstruction or arteriolar dilatation. For example, histamine relaxes the smooth muscle of the arterioles. When present in large amounts, histamine constricts the venules. Therefore, the capillary pressure is increased and an abnormal amount of fluid flows from the vascular to the interstitial compartment.

Due to vasodilation during tissue activity, larger quantities of fluid pass out of the capillaries into the interstitial compartment. During muscular exercise, the weight of the muscle may be increased by 20 per cent. This increased amount of tissue fluid supplies the active organs with more oxygen, nutrients, water, electrolytes, and hormones necessary for carrying out the specific functions of these organs.

The role of the arterioles in capillary hydrostatic pressure. The arterioles control the amount of blood entering the capillaries, thus determining the hydrostatic pressure within the capillaries. An increased arteriolar resistance (vasoconstriction) leads to a decreased capillary pressure. In acute conditions, vasoconstriction preserves blood flow in certain visceral organs at the expense of the periphery.

A decreased arteriolar resistance (vasodilatation) leads to an increased capillary pressure. Hence, to connect knowledge, increased vasomotor stimulation of the arterioles (as occurs initially in shock) causes an intense arteriolar constriction. Consequently, there is a decreased hydrostatic pressure and a decreased amount of the five substances crossing the capillary membrane into the interstitial compartment. The cells are then deprived of sufficient amounts of the five substances. This leads to anaerobic metabolism with a consequent de-

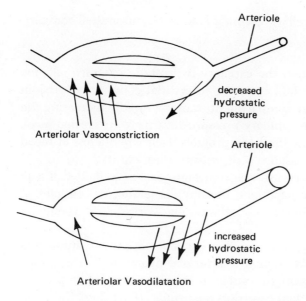

Figure 10. Above. *Arteriolar vasoconstriction.* Below. *Arteriolar vasodilatation.*

creased cell metabolism and energy formation, hence the weakness of the four types of cells: muscle, nerve, connective, and epithelial. However prostrating this may be, the intense arteriolar resistance plays a vital role to increase the circulating blood volume. As mentioned previously, normally, small proteins are forced across the capillary membrane by hydrostatic pressure. If this hydrostatic pressure is decreased, as it is in arteriolar vasoconstriction, then these small proteins remain in the capillary blood stream, pass to the venous end of the capillary and enhance the colloid osmotic pressure which, in turn, pulls a greater amount of fluid from the interstitial compartment into the vascular compartment to increase the blood volume. This is an extremely important mechanism that occurs in the initial stage of hemorrhagic shock to protect the body. Important implications for nursing care derive from this.

Initially, the diastolic blood pressure, at the time of arteriolar constriction, will be elevated over normal because, among other things, the diastolic blood pressure is a measure of peripheral arteriolar resistance, or vasoconstriction. The systolic blood pressure will be maintained fairly close to normal (unless the amount of blood loss is rapid and severe) because of the increased venous return, due, in part, to the large remobilization of fluid from the interstitial compartment, and, in part, to the constriction of the veins. Continuous bleeding, without adequate treatment, will lead to decreased systolic and diastolic pressures.

In many instances, peripheral arteriolar constriction is eventually replaced by arteriolar dilatation. When this occurs, the hydrostatic pressure of the blood entering the capillaries is increased markedly, and vast amounts of fluid are forced across the capillary membrane into the interstitial compartment. The circulating blood volume, as a consequence, decreases drastically, and, because of the passage of more proteins than normal into the interstitial compartment from the arteriolar end of the capillary, the colloid osmotic pressure increases in the interstitial compartment. Therefore, excess fluids are held in the interstitial compartment. Because of the decreased protein content at the venous end of the capillary, the colloid osmotic pressure will be decreased there, resulting in a decreased ability to pull fluid into the capillary. Excess fluid and wastes in the interstitial compartment results in edema and metabolic acidosis.

The venules and veins

As mentioned earlier, it is at the venous end of the capillary that excess fluids are normally pulled out of the interstitial compartment by osmosis. Although the arterioles are referred to as the *resistance* vessels, the veins are called the *capacitance* vessels; meaning that they can hold large volumes of blood. Anatomically, the layers of the veins are much thinner than those of the arteries and arterioles; therefore, the veins are much more distensible.

Venous resistance. Although the veins are noted mainly for their capacitance, they, like the arteries and arterioles, are also innervated by the sympathetic vasomotor nerves. Because the layers of the veins are thinner than the arterial layers, the extent to which veins can constrict is much less than the arterioles. When the veins constrict, there is a decrease in the total capacity of the venous system. The decreased venous capacity forces the blood toward the right side of the heart. There is, therefore, an increase in venous flow and an increase in venous pressure. Venous constriction raises venous pressure just as arteriolar constriction raises arterial pressure. The greater the venous pressure, the greater is the capillary pressure; hence there is a resistance to blood flow out of the capillaries into the veins. In the

55

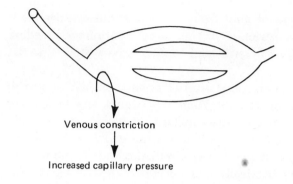

Venous constriction

Increased capillary pressure

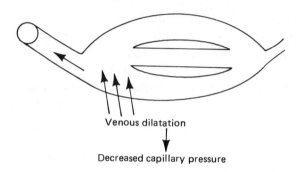

Venous dilatation

Decreased capillary pressure

Figure 11. Above. *Venous constriction.* Below. *Venous dilatation.*

initial stage of hemorrhagic shock, this increased return of blood to the heart will lead to a greater cardiac output from the left ventricle. Considering that about 70 per cent of all the blood in the circulatory circuit is in the systemic veins, the term "venous reservoir" is often used. Marked venous dilatation, e.g., in the warm phase of septic shock, can cause blood to pool in the veins, thereby decreasing the flow of blood to the right heart and, consequently, decreasing the cardiac output.

The venous plexuses of the entire body, including those of the hands, feet, arms, and trunk are supplied with sympathetic vasoconstrictor nerves. In times of circulatory stress, e.g., as results from excessive exercise, hemorrhage, or states of anxiety, these vasoexcitor nerves are stimulated—the result of which is vasoconstriction of the peripheral veins, as well as the arterioles, in the area.

Effect of venous resistance on the capillary. An increased venous resistance (constriction) leads to an increased capillary pressure. A decreased venous resistance (dilatation) leads to a decreased capillary pressure. Study Fig. 11 carefully. Vasoconstrictor drugs must always be given with extreme caution. The administration of such drugs causes arteriolar *and* venous constriction. Therefore, less blood enters the capillary at the arteriolar end (increased arteriolar resistance leads to decreased capillary pressure). After initial venous constriction, which squeezes and propels blood rapidly from the veins to the right atrium, the capillary pressure increases and plasma fluid is forced from the capillaries into the interstitial compartment, thus decreasing the circulating blood volume. Consequently, the return of venous blood to the right atrium will be drastically reduced. This means, of course, that cardiac output will also be drastically reduced. Thus it can be seen that veins, as well as arterioles, play a big role in capillary dynamics.

The role of carbon dioxide in circulatory dynamics

PRINCIPLE 20: There is a direct relationship between metabolism and carbon dioxide production; as metabolism increases, the amount of carbon dioxide produced by the tissues increases.

PRINCIPLE 21: There is a direct relationship between metabolism and the amount of blood required by the tissues; when metabolism increases, the blood flow is correspondingly increased.

Carbon dioxide acts locally upon the walls of the veins and exerts a dilator effect. On the other hand, a decrease in carbon dioxide produces venous constriction and so interferes with the return of blood to the heart. Breathing an air mixture rich in carbon dioxide relaxes the smaller veins and causes an improved flow of venous blood back to the right side of the heart.

Viscosity of venous blood. Because of the decreased oxygen content in venous blood, venous blood is more viscous than arterial blood.

Venous valves. In general, veins greater than 1 mm. in diameter are equipped with valves, affording little interference with the return of blood to the heart and preventing a reversal of blood flow. Valves are most numerous in the veins of the lower extremities; they are absent in the venae cavae, the veins of the intestine, and the brain.

57

Distribution of veins

Veins usually accompany arteries, however, there are certain points of difference:

1. Veins are distributed in two sets: superficial and deep.
2. Blood from the digestive tract is returned by a special system of vessels; the portal system. The blood from the portal system is returned to the inferior vena cava through the hepatic veins.
3. Whereas blood flows through only *one* artery (aorta) in leaving the heart, *three* veins return the blood to the heart. They are the coronary sinus draining the coronary veins of the heart; the superior vena cava draining the head, neck, thorax, and upper extremities; and the inferior vena cava draining the lower part of the body.

The venous pump

In contrast to the flow of arterial blood, which is forcefully pumped out of the left ventricle, the venous flow towards the right side of the heart is not aided by the pumping action of the heart. How, then, does venous blood flow into the right atrium? This is accomplished by the so-called *venous pump*, which consists of the following mechanisms:

1. The movement and tenseness of the leg muscles propels venous blood toward the right atrium, thereby decreasing the venous pressure in the dependent veins. The venous pressure in the feet of a walking person is less than 25 mm/Hg. If the person stands still, the venous pressure in the feet will rise to 90 mm. Hg. in about 30 seconds. As a consequence, the capillary pressure will also rise and plasma fluid will leak from the capillaries into the interstitial compartment, causing edema and a decreased circulating blood volume. As much as 15 to 20 per cent of the blood volume can be lost from the circulation within the first 15 minutes of quiet standing.
2. The valves in the peripheral veins prevent the back-flow of blood; hence, the venous blood can move only in one direction.
3. The pumping action of the diaphragm (the thoracic pump) propels venous blood toward the right side of the heart.
4. Negative intrathoracic pressure: since fluids flow from an area of greater to lesser points of pressure, the flow of the venous blood is upward toward the lesser point of pressure. Any disor-

der of any of these four mechanisms will result in a decreased return of venous blood to the right atrium. Among such disorders are:

a. Inactivity or prolonged bedrest
b. Nonfunctioning valves, as in varicose veins
c. Shallow breathing or diaphragmatic hernias
d. An increased intrathoracic pressure due to the Valsalva maneuver or a pneumothorax.

Venous pressure and central venous pressure (CVP)

"Venous pressure" is the force exerted by the blood on the walls of the veins. Unlike the arterial pressure, which is greatest in the aorta, venous pressure is greatest in the lower extremities. On standing, the pressure in the neck veins falls so low that the atmospheric pressure on the outside of the neck causes them to collapse. Distended neck veins in a sitting or standing position is indicative of an elevated venous pressure. Pulsation of the neck veins, while sitting, indicates that the venous pressure is markedly elevated.

Venous pressure arises primarily from the arterial pressure which is transmitted through the capillary bed. One can obtain a cursory evaluation of the venous pressure by observing the peripheral veins of the hand. Normally, when the hand is elevated, the veins empty in 3 to 5 seconds. When the hand is lowered, the veins fill in 3 to 5 seconds. During early stages of shock, there is slow emptying and filling of these veins.

As the venous pump propels the blood upward toward the right side of the heart, the venous pressure decreases gradually, until it becomes zero above the level of the tricuspid valve in the right atrium. This is referred to as *central venous pressure*.

Normal Pulmonary Circulation and Implications of the Abnormal

For a complete understanding of central venous pressure, it is necessary to review the normal circulation of blood from the right atrium to the left ventricle. Venous blood enters the right atrium from the venae cavae, is pumped from the right atrium to the right ventricle, goes through the pulmonary artery to the capillary blood stream of the lungs where carbon dioxide and oxygen exchange, by diffusion, in the alveoli. Fresh oxygenated blood then flows via the four pulmonary veins to the left atrium, to the left ventricle, and then out through the aorta. If there were a weakness in any part of the myocardium, it is obvious that blood would not adequately be pumped out of the respective chamber; hence, the pressure of the blood would increase there and would be reflected backward along the circuit. For example, with left myocardial failure, blood would not be forced out of the left ventricle in normal amounts. Consequently, blood in the left atrium, pulmonary veins, pulmonary capillary blood stream, pulmonary artery, right ventricle, and right atrium would reflect an increased pressure. Since the normal right atrial pressure is zero, the pressure there would be increased with myocardial weakness, or failure. Initially, the right side of the heart maintains its pumping power, even though the left side may be in failure; therefore, right atrial pressure may stay close to normal for quite awhile. This means, then, that the increased pressure would be reflected in the pulmonary capillary blood stream. In fact, a strong right myocardium would only add insult to injury, as it would continue to pump blood to the lungs while the pressure within the pulmonary capillary blood stream is increasing, due to the incomplete emptying. In this instance, the bulk of the backward pressure would be reflected in the pulmonary circuit. Since the alveolar membrane is extremely thin, and fluids flow to an area of least resistance, plasma fluid is forced into the alveoli. As a result, the alveolar surface area for the diffusion of gases is decreased, and the patient experiences shortness of breath. If left myocardial contractility is not strengthened, thus relieving the back pressure, the patient will literally drown in his own fluid.

MONITORING THE CENTRAL VENOUS PRESSURE

"Today, with a myriad of instruments, we can explore things we never imagined. But we no longer *see* what is right in front of us."
—*Thomas Merton,* Conjectures of a Guilty Bystander (from *TIME,* Aug. 5, 1966, p 73).

The central venous pressure represents right atrial pressure and is determined by a complex interaction of blood volume, cardiac pump action, and vascular tone alterations. Monitoring of the CVP is helpful in the management of patients in circulatory failure, as it reflects the dynamic interrelationship between these three components. Since shock represents a failure of any one or more of these three mechanisms, CVP monitoring is useful in the diagnosis and treatment of patients in shock. The primary concern should be to maintain adequate circulation as reflected by the patient's general appearance: color and temperature of the skin and mucous membranes, quality of the pulse, urine output, and arterial blood pressure.

Central venous pressure indicates the difference between venous return to the right atrium and right ventricular output. Increases in right atrial pressure reflect increases in right ventricular diastolic pressure, a sign of right heart failure. CVP does *not* accurately reflect blood volume, per se, rather, it indicates the relationship between the blood volume which enters the right atrium and the effectiveness of the right ventricle to eject that volume into the pulmonary artery. The CVP is measured in the right atrium (the normal is 0–4 Cm. water), or the superior vena cava (the normal is 6–8 Cm. water). It is primarily a reflection of ventricular filling pressure, and, therefore, of ventricular competence. An increase in right atrial pressure reflects an increase in right ventricular diastolic pressure.

CVP as a guide to the state of left ventricular function is probably without justification, and could result in greater hazard than benefit.

ALTERATIONS OF THE CENTRAL VENOUS PRESSURE

1. When cardiac pump action and vascular tone are stable, the CVP will vary directly with alterations in the blood volume. CVP monitoring is indicated during acute circulatory failure when it is difficult to stablize circulatory dynamics, and the relationship of the blood volume to cardiac pump capacity is not certain. CVP does not accurately reflect the blood volume, but it is a useful indicator of the competence of the heart to accept and expel the blood returned to it. Because of this, CVP is an excellent guide to safe volume repletion. As such, it reflects cardiac competency in handling the blood volume.

CVP is essential in diagnosing and correcting deficits of blood volume and, to a lesser degree, in evaluating myocardial insufficiency. In general, a rising CVP around 17 Cm. water indicates a blood volume and venous return which are close to the limit that can be managed by the myocardium at that time. Further fluid replacement is not likely to produce a favorable response until the heart action is improved. Some physicians are of the opinion that volume replacement can be pursued with reasonable safety if the CVP is maintained below

15 Cm. water. When replacement therapy has been pushed to this point, but without achieving restoration of the blood pressure and general patient-improvement, a cardiac deficit must be present.

The greatest value of CVP is to enable a vigorous replacement of fluids to the maximum extent, while at the same time minimizing pulmonary edema. A CVP of 0–5 Cm. water (when the catheter is in the superior vena cava) indicates hypovolemia and a need for intravenous fluid therapy. If the CVP goes above 12 Cm. water, either fluid overloading or myocardial failure may be present. If the CVP goes beyond 14 Cm. water, pulmonary edema will most likely occur. Pulmonary edema results when the pulmonary capillary hydrostatic pressure exceeds the pulmonary colloid osmotic pressure. If the heart is in failure, increased CVP measurements and pulmonary rales will promptly indicate this, as well as the risk of infusing additional fluids.

The effect of fluid replacement on the patient in shock should be gauged by changes which reflect circulatory competence, such as blood pressure, mental acuity, urinary output, peripheral venous filling, and color, temperature, and texture of the skin. Elevation of the CVP without improvement of the arterial blood pressure and urinary output would be indicative of circulatory failure.

2. When blood volume and vascular tone are stable, the CVP will vary *inversely* with right cardiac pump action. If the right heart fails to pump efficiently, the CVP will increase. (With frank left ventricular failure, however, a rise in CVP may be delayed as long as the right ventricle remains competent.) As the heart is strengthened, the CVP will decrease toward normal.

It should be pointed out that an elevated CVP does not always contraindicate blood replacement. Circulatory collapse can lead to inadequate coronary perfusion, which, of itself, can account for myocardial failure. If cardiac failure is due to inadequate coronary perfusion, it is best treated by volume replacement with close supervision of the CVP during the infusion. As the coronary flow improves, the myocardium will become stronger and the CVP will decrease.

3. Changes in vascular tone may affect the CVP independently. Any factor which reduces the return of blood to the heart, such as decreased venous tone (dilatation), and arteriolar vasoconstriction, will tend to decrease the CVP.

Anything that causes a rapid inflow of venous blood into the right atrium tends to increase the CVP. Some of the factors which increase the venous return of blood are:

a. Increased blood volume
b. Increased venous tone (venous constriction)
c. Arteriolar dilatation.

Increases in CVP are also characteristic of pulmonary embolization. This rise is often accompanied by signs of respiratory distress and rales, which are indicative of pulmonary edema. Caution should be used in giving fluids, as the blood volume may already be normal, and the circulatory circuit could become overloaded. Sympathomimetics (vasoconstrictors) are indicated, with no additional fluids.

PROCEDURE

An intracatheter is inserted by the physician and passed into the superior vena cava via the subclavian vein, infraclavicularly, or into the right atrium, and is connected to a manometer. The procedure may also be done supraclavicularly, or via the external or internal jugular vein. The normal pressure in the right atrium is zero, and in the superior vena cava it is 6–8 Cm. water.

When checking a patient's CVP, the zero mark on the manometer should be at the same level as the patient's right atrium. Usually, the CVP is checked with the patient lying in a supine position. The mid-axillary line should be marked, and the zero point on the manometer should be placed exactly at this mark. The manometer should be held at a right angle. All subsequent readings should be taken with the patient in the same position. A written record should be kept of the CVP readings.

Complications that can arise

Extreme caution must be taken that the intracatheter line does not become disengaged from the intravenous line and stopcock. Should this occur, air will be sucked into the line, due to the negative intrathoracic pressure. This, of course, could result in an air embolus and possible death.

Since there is danger of a pneumothorax following subclavian cannulation, the nurse should observe the patient for signs and symptoms.

Other uses for CVP catheterization

Besides the measurements of central venous pressure, CVP catheterization can also be used for the following:

1. Blood phlebotomy
2. Recordings of atrial electrograms
3. Securing blood samples for laboratory analysis
4. Administering drugs
5. Hyperalimentation fluids

Estimation of the central venous pressure without an intracatheter

In the absence of a CVP manometer, the venous pressure can often be estimated by simply observing for any distension of the peripheral veins, especially the neck veins. When the right atrial pressure becomes increased to as much as 13 Cm. water, the lower veins of the neck begin to distend, even when in a sitting position. Normally, in a sitting position, the neck veins are not distended. A rough estimate of the venous pressure can be made while observing the distension of the antecubital or hand veins. As the arm is progressively raised, the veins will collapse suddenly. The level at which they collapse is a rough measure of the venous pressure. In severe cardiac failure, the venous pressure increases markedly, and one can usually detect pulsation in the neck veins. This is an important diagnostic sign of severe congestive heart failure.

False readings of the central venous pressure

The following might give false high CVP readings:

1. Coughing
2. Positive pressure breathing
3. Abdominal distension
4. Cardiac tamponade
5. Obstruction of the outlet of the right ventricle, or great vessels distal to the position of the catheter
6. Pneumothorax
7. Changes in posture

The CVP may be falsely low in patients with airway obstruction during inspiration, during assisted ventilation with negative pressure cycling, and in changes in body posture.

PULMONARY ARTERY WEDGE PRESSURE (PAWP OR PWP)

Considering that the heart consists of *two* pumps—the right and the left—reflections of the effectiveness of each pump is desirable.

Although the CVP reflects the right atrial pressure, it is not a practical reflection of left atrial pressure. Patients with gross fluid overload, even with marked pulmonary edema, often have a normal CVP. In other words the left heart can be in severe failure, while the right heart can continue to pump effectively for awhile and reflect a low CVP.

Something further was needed to measure the left atrial pressure, in order to ensure expeditious treatment. Thus evolved the use of the Swan-Ganz Catheter to measure the pulmonary artery end diastolic pressure or pulmonary artery wedge pressure. The Swan-Ganz monitor of pulmonary capillary wedge pressure is an excellent device for recording left atrial pressure; hence, left ventricular diastolic filling pressure.

Pulmonary artery wedge pressures are presently preferred over central venous pressure in monitoring left ventricular filling pressure. A Swan-Ganz catheter is usually inserted into an antecubital vein and threaded through to a thoracic vein, or it can be inserted into a subclavian vessel. Blood flow carries the ballooned catheter into the right atrium, through the tricuspid valve, into the right ventricle, and up the main pulmonary artery.* The catheter can be floated up and wedged in a branch of the pulmonary artery. Hence, the term pulmonary capillary "wedge" pressure (PCWP). The catheter records the pressure transmitted back across the pulmonary capillary bed from the pulmonary veins. The mean pulmonary capillary pressure is approximately 7 mm. Hg. The catheter is often left in place for periods up to one week. Periodically, the balloon can be inflated to obtain the measurements of the pulmonary artery wedge pressure. Constant inflation of the balloon could lead to pulmonary infarction and segmental ischemia.

The pulmonary artery diastolic and pulmonary capillary wedge pressures reflect left ventricular end diastolic pressure (LVEDP), which is the pressure in the left ventricle immediately preceding contraction. In a normal person, the pressure before contraction of the left heart should be equal to the pressure in the pulmonary artery and pulmonary capillaries. Hence, left heart failure, as well as an increased or decreased blood volume can be detected in the pressure readings.

Perhaps the benefit of pulmonary wedge pressure is that increases in pressure can be detected *before* insipient signs and symptoms of

---

* The normal diastolic pulmonary artery pressure is approximately 8 mm. Hg., and the mean pulmonary artery pressure is about 13 mm. Hg.

left heart failure or fluid-overload occur. In contrast to CVP, this is a marked asset, as CVP readings may be within the normal range while the left ventricle is failing.

Cardiogenic shock and pulmonary wedge pressure

In cardiogenic shock due to left heart failure, the PAWP readings will be elevated over normal. Pulmonary artery wedge pressure provides two important assets in the management of the patient in cardiogenic shock: (1) it is a reliable means of assessing left ventricular preload, which is of importance in determining the performance of the heart, and (2) it is a reliable indicator in assessing pulmonary capillary pressure, which is a determinant of pulmonary edema. For example, if the PWP is greater than 17 mm/Hg., pulmonary congestion can occur. Alveolar pulmonary edema can occur when the wedge pressure exceeds 25 mm. Hg. According to Evans, "The objective in cardiogenic shock is to add volume, if necessary, to elevate the pulmonary artery end diastolic pressure (PAEDP), keeping it less than 20 mm. Hg., which is high enough to obtain the best cardiac output, but low enough to avoid development of pulmonary edema."[4] As stated earlier, whether or not edema forms is dependent on the difference between capillary hydrostatic pressure and plasma colloid osmotic pressure. For this reason, colloid osmotic/hydrostatic pressure gradients are often measured.

THE VALSALVA MANEUVER AND ITS IMPLICATIONS

Definition: A sustained increase in intrathoracic pressure caused by straining or blowing against some resistance for 20 to 30 seconds. Forced expiratory effort against a closed glottis.

PRINCIPLE 22: The movement of fluids from one area to another is dependent upon a difference in pressure at both ends.
PRINCIPLE 23: Fluids flow from areas of greater to lesser points of pressure.
PRINCIPLE 24: There is an inverse relationship between the intrathoracic pressure and the return of venous blood to the right atrium.
    a. An increased intrathoracic pressure leads to a decreased return of venous blood to the right atrium.

[4] Roger, Evans, "Cardiogenic Shock: Can the Prognosis be Improved?" *Postgraduate Medicine*, **58** (Dec. 1975), p. 81.

b. A decreased intrathoracic pressure leads to an increased return of venous blood to the right atrium.

Normally, blood flows back to the right atrium via the inferior and superior venae cavae. If the left side of the heart can only pump out the amount of blood that flows into the right side of the heart, then it will follow that a decreased venous return to the right atrium will lead to a decreased cardiac output from the left ventricle, with a subsequent decreased flow through the coronary artery to the myocardium, as well as to *all* body parts.

A decreased venous return to the right atrium is a direct consequence of the Valsalva maneuver, which is characterized by an increased intrathoracic pressure. Normally, at the end of inspiration, the intrapleural pressure (between the visceral and parietal pleurae) becomes more negative, and air is pulled into the lungs. On expiration, the elastic recoil of the alveoli and the upward movement of the diaphragm push air out of the lungs to the atmosphere. Upon straining, or holding the breath after an inspiration, there is an expiratory effort against a closed glottis and air is not released to the atmosphere. This creates compression of the lungs with a subsequent increased intrathoracic pressure.

Anything that increases the intrathoracic pressure can cause decreased venous return, decreased cardiac output, decreased systolic blood pressure, and reflex sympathetic impulses from the vasomotor center that lead to arteriolar vasoconstriction of the fingers, toes, and calf muscles. There is also a decreased return of blood from the head and legs. Decreased flow of blood from the head can lead to increased intracranial pressure, decreased systolic blood pressure, and reflex tachycardia. The increased intracranial pressure is due to the retention of blood in the vessels of the brain. In turn, this can lead to a relative degree of cerebral hypoxia. Since the perfusion pressure of the brain is the difference between intracranial pressure and mean systemic arterial blood pressure, the perfusion pressure will be decreased and hypoxia of the brain cells may easily occur. During straining, there is a marked increase in CVP, presumably due to the decreased cardiac output. When the straining ceases, blood rushes into the thorax and the resurgent cardiac output is thrust into the arterial blood vessels which are constricted. This results in a brief overshoot of the arterial blood pressure. As the blood pressure increases, an opposite reflex adjustment occurs in the slowing of the heart rate (bradycardia), and pressures to prestrain levels. According to Sodeman and Sodeman, in heart failure, the blood pressure actually increases during straining and the overshoot in arterial pressure and reflex bradycardia do not occur.[5]

Factors predisposing to increased intrathoracic pressure

Anything that increases the intrathoracic pressure can cause a decrease in venous return, decreased cardiac output, and an increased intracranial pressure. Obviously, there should not be any interference with the thoracic pump and the normal breathing process. Yet, and unwittingly, in many instances of nursing care and treatment, this *does* occur.

Very forceful coughing, and energetic straining, such as occurs with straining at stool during constipation, causes extreme elevations in intrathoracic and intra-abdominal pressures which may rise as high as 200 mm. Hg. Although the Valsalva maneuver has little effect on the respiratory structures, per se, it causes striking effects on the circulation. Patients with coronary artery disease or cerebral vascular accidents should be instructed against vigorous coughing and straining.

Since it is an increased intrathoracic pressure that causes the Valsalva maneuver, measures should be taken to avoid this. Anything that causes the patient to strain or hold his breath against a closed glottis will impede the flow of blood into the right atrium. For example, when assisting a patient up in bed, who among us has not said, "All right, when I count to three, push and I'll scoot you up in bed. One . . . two . . . three." On the count of three, the patient usually will hold his breath and close his glottis. This will cause the Valsalva maneuver. The same can occur while turning a patient in bed, making the bed, assisting him to sit up in bed, arousing him from sleep, manipulating a painful limb, or reaching for an overhead trapeze bar. In addition, prolonged suctioning over 12 seconds, the prone (face down) position, or extreme flexion of the hips or neck can also cause the Valsalva maneuver. Although the intrathoracic pressure increase may be transient, there may not be any harmful effects, but there *could* be; these effects would be due to a decreased venous return, a decreased cardiac output, or increased intracranial pressure, or a combination of these. Depending on the age and physical condition of the patient, he may faint, he may have a cerebral vascular accident, or he may die because

---

[5] William A. Sodeman, and William A. Sodeman, Jr., *Pathologic Physiology*, 5th ed., Philadelphia: W. B. Saunders Co., 1974, pp. 186–187.

of decreased cardiac output. The vulnerable heart patient could die suddenly, due to decreased coronary perfusion.

When one strains to pass stool, the breath is held, the glottis is closed, and the diaphragm is fixed downward resulting in a markedly reduced venous inflow to the right heart. Constipation exaggerates this, as a person might strain several times within a short span of time. According to Burton, "Even in the normal posture in the bathroom, the act of defecation, accompanied by the Valsalva maneuver, can impose a severe load on the heart. Cardiac patients often die at stool. The effort of trying to defecate in the supine position can put an even greater burden on the heart. Ban the bedpan!"[6]

Many more examples of causes of the Valsalva maneuver could be given, such as micturition, some forms of isometric exercises, bearing down during the delivery process, positive pressure breathing, shoveling snow, and so on. According to Secor, "In patients with poor circulation, intermittent positive pressure breathing (IPPB) may cause circulatory collapse due to impaired venous return to the heart and decreased cardiac output, a condition that is reversed when the positive pressure is reduced."[7]

How to prevent the valsalva maneuver

There are marked indications for teaching both the sick and the well. Merely instructing the patient to continue to breathe normally, not to hold his breath, will greatly decrease the incidence of the Valsalva maneuver. It is hoped that there will be nursing research in the near future to study the effects of other basic nursing care measures on venous inflow to the heart.

It is obvious that the prevention of the Valsalva maneuver in the shock patient is imperative. Whether shock is due to heart failure, loss of blood volume, or vasodilatation, the patient's tolerance to the Valsalva Maneuver would be severely decreased.

REFERENCES

Baker, Robert J. "Monitoring in Critically Ill Patients." *Surgical Clinics of North America,* **57,** (Dec. 1977), 1139–1158.
Beland, Irene L. *Clinical Nursing.* 2nd ed. New York: Macmillan Publishing Co., Inc., 1970.

[6] Burton, op. cit., p. 166.
[7] Secor, op. cit., p. 127.

Chaffee, Ellen E., and Esther M. Greisheimer. *Basic Physiology and Anatomy.* 3rd ed. Philadelphia: J. B. Lippincott Co., 1974.

da Luz, P. L., M. H. Weil, and H. Shubin. "Current Concepts on Mechanics and Treatment of Cardiogenic Shock." *American Heart Journal,* 92 (July 1976).

Gunnar, R. M., H. S. Loeb, S. A. Johnson, and P. J. Scanlon. "Cardiovascular Assist Devices in Cardiogenic Shock." *Journal of the American Medical Association,* 236 (Oct. 4, 1976), 1614–1621.

Guyton, Arthur C. *Medical Physiology.* 5th ed. Philadelphia: W. B. Saunders Co., 1976.

Hadley, Florence, and Katherine J. Bordicks. "When a Patient Has Respiratory Difficulty." *American Journal of Nursing,* 62 (Oct. 1962), 64–67.

MacLean, L. D., Duff, J. H., Scott, H. M., and D. W. Peretz. Treatment of Shock in Man Based on Hemodynamic Diagnosis. *Surgery, Gynecology, and Obstetrics* 120:1 (1965).

Mauss, N. K., and P. H. Mitchell. "Increased Intracranial Pressure: An Update." *Heart and Lung,* 5 (Nov.–Dec. 1976), 919–926.

Murray, J., and J. Smallwood. "CVP Monitoring." *Nursing '77* (Jan. 1977), 42–47.

Rau, J., and M. Rau. "To Breathe or Be Breathed, Understanding I.P.P.B." *American Journal of Nursing,* 77, (April 1977), 613–617.

Scanlon, P. J. "Cardiovascular Assist Devices in Cardiogenic Shock." *Journal of the American Medical Association,* 236 (Oct. 4, 1976), 1619–1621.

Woods, Susan L. "Monitoring Pulmonary Artery Pressures." *American Journal of Nursing* (Nov. 1976), 1765–1771.

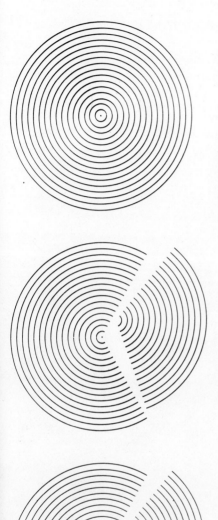

PART II

Health, Disease, Stress, and Adaptation

CHAPTER 5

Health and Disease

Man's Purpose

No matter how significant or insignificant he may appear, man is two things:

1. He is a living, thinking spirit, whose presence on this earth is to fulfill a Divine purpose, and
2. He is a magnificent machine whose parts, in health, are in tune for the purpose of protecting and sustaining his life.

The nurse's overall purpose for being is to care for the ill (the patients whose bodies are out of tune) and to assist them back to as balanced and optimal a state of health as is possible. By doing this, she will be helping to prolong lives, thereby assisting human beings to fulfill their purposes. As Sr. Vaillot has so aptly said, "The nursing process is called into being by a dysfunction in the patient's homeostatic condition. She should help the patient either to reduce the stress or to reinforce his ability to cope with it, or both."[1]

[1] Madeleine Clemence Vaillot, Sr. "Nursing Theory, Levels of Nursing, and Curriculum Development," *Nursing Forum* IX (1970), 234–249.

Health (Homeostasis) and Disease

"Health is a state of complete physical, mental, and social well-being, and not merely the absence of disease and infirmity."[2]

Health should not be taken for granted. The nurse must possess an understanding and appreciation of *health* before she can fully understand her role in caring for the sick. She must realize that illness is accompanied by dependence on her. Indeed, is this not her reason for being?

A Comprehensive Theory of Disease

The organism is only a living machine constructed in such a fashion that, on the one hand, there is full communication between the external environment and the milieu interieur, and on the other, there are protective functions of organic elements holding living materials in reserve and maintaining without interruption humidity, heat, and other conditions indispensable to vital activity. Sickness and death are only dislocations or perturbations of that mechanism. (Claude Bernard, from *Introduction a l'Etude de la Medicine Experimental,* 1895.)

PRINCIPLE 25: A state of health implies a dynamic equilibrium of the body and its parts—homeostasis.

The most comprehensive generalization of physiology is that the body reacts to environmental changes (internal or external) in such a way as to preserve the integrity of the whole organism and of its constituent parts. Homeostasis is synonymous with health. Dr. Bernard said that one of the greatest characteristics of all living beings is their ability to maintain a constancy of their internal environment. This constancy of the internal environment was later termed *homeostasis* by Dr. Walter B. Cannon.[3] Among other things, the body's homeostatic mechanisms are directed toward maintaining a dynamic equilibrium of osmotic pressure. Therefore, it is not surprising that severe dehydration is associated with severe electrolyte imbalance. The same is true for overhydration, i.e., water-intoxication.

The normal act of perspiring helps to maintain an internal balance

[2] United Nations World Health Organization. Secondary Source: Kay Corman Kintzel (ed.). *Advanced Concepts in Clinical Nursing,* Philadelphia: J. B. Lippincott Co., 1971, p. 21.
[3] Walter B. Cannon. *The Wisdom of the Body,* New York: Norton, 1939.

by preventing the internal environment from becoming overheated. Or, we might consider a house which is thermostatically controlled to maintain a constant temperature of 70 degrees, despite changing temperatures outside the house. *Thermostasis* means the maintenance of a steady temperature, and, like homeostasis, it is self-regulated. Whenever this self-regulating power fails, either disease or death ensues.

Health implies a state of dynamic balance, and since neither we nor our environment is static, in health there is a constantly shifting balance, a state of *dynamic* equilibrium. The healthy body is able to meet its changing needs. The example of perspiring applies, as do many others. For instance, when one runs, the heart is stimulated to pump faster, thus pumping additional quantities of blood to those muscles needing it most. This is another example of how the healthy body adapts to meet its changing needs.

Recently, it has been suggested by Heilbrunn that "biostasis" is a more general term that includes "All the phenomena in which living organisms resist changes in their environment, in which they tend to preserve their constancy."[4]

DISEASE

"In the medicine of the future, it is likely that we will pay more and more attention to homeostatic aspects of the individual with the goal that we will recognize disease and control it in its incipient form before the body's autoregulative mechanisms have been pushed to the breaking point."[5]

Hippocrates, the Father of Medicine, said that disease is not only suffering but also toil, i.e., a fight of the body to restore itself toward normal. He said that there is a healing force of nature which cures from within. Disease, then, is not mere surrender, but it is a fight for health, and unless there is fight, there is no disease.[6]

Not every deviation from normal is disease. For instance, a man who has lost an arm or leg is not ill for the rest of his life. He may be in perfect health, despite his physical handicap. No longer is his body fighting to restore a diseased arm or leg to health. The concept

[4] Howard C. Hopps. Principles of Pathology, New York: Appleton-Century-Crofts, 1964, p. 3.
[5] Ibid, p. 4.
[6] Hans Selye. The Stress of Life, Revised Ed., New York: McGraw-Hill Book Co., 1976, p. 11.

of disease presupposes a clash between forces of aggression and our defenses.[7]

In a state of health the body is able to meet its changing needs. Shock is due to a breakdown of the body's defense mechanisms.

In early shock, the body valiantly strives to protect itself by maintaining a balanced state, and it does, for awhile, by using its reserve forces—its compensatory or adaptive mechanisms. In actuality, the signs and symptoms exhibited by the patient in early shock are evidence of his compensatory forces at work. In the advanced stage of shock, however, the body's reserves become exhausted and depleted, and the ability to adapt and to fight an aggressor decreases. It is at this point, when the body has exhausted its ability to protect itself, that the major signs and symptoms of shock become manifest. The body tissues, as a consequence, suffer from an inadequate supply of blood; hence there is a decrease of oxygen, nutrients, water, electrolytes, and hormones to all body cells. Cellular hypoxia results, as well as the accumulation of cellular acid waste products. As a result, there is a subsequent dysfunction of the cells, tissues, organs, and systems, along with increasing metabolic acidosis.

[7] Ibid, p. 12.

CHAPTER 6

Stress and Adaptation

Stress

PRINCIPLE 26:   Adaptation is basic to survival.

The tensions of responsibility do not necessarily shorten a man's life. Stress cannot be measured or described by the external circumstances with which a man must contend, but rather by his *reaction* to these circumstances. One man's stress may be another man's pleasure.[1]

Stress can either cure or aggravate a disease. Stress represents a pattern of physiological reactions that prepare a person for action. In that sense, stress enables man to survive in a hostile environment.[2]

The notion of socially-induced stress as a precipitating factor in chronic diseases is gaining acceptance among a wide spectrum of scientists. It is becoming recognized that stress can be one of the components of *any* disease, not just of those designated as "psychosomatic."[3]

[1] Sidney Pell and C. Anthony D'Alonzo. *Time* (Sept. 27, 1963), p. 62.
[2] Hans Selye. The Stress of Life, 8th Ed., New York: McGraw-Hill Book Co., 1956, p. 156.
[3] Judith G. Rabkin and Elmer L. Struening. "Life Events, Stress, and Illness," *Science*, **194** (Dec. 1976), 1014.

Stress can be controlled in either of two ways: by manipulating the *nature* of man, himself, or by controlling his environment.

To facilitate the reader's understanding of stress and stressors to be presented in the following paragraphs, an analogy from everyday life will be presented.

If a man loses his job, he uses his unemployment insurance and savings to tide him over until he gets another job. When these are exhausted, he might receive help from his relatives and friends. If he has neither relatives nor friends, he has to find other means until he is able to renew his resources. If he does not find other means, or another job, he will be exposed to hunger. The stressor is the loss of the man's job. His savings and any assistance he may have received from relatives and friends can be considered as stress reactions, as they are compensatory, or adaptive mechanisms. Finally, exhaustion of all monetary resources (loss of compensatory, adaptive mechanisms) leads to hunger, which is a direct result of his inability to adapt. Keep this analogy in mind.

Stressors and Stress

Selye defines a *stressor* as anything that produces stress, thus constituting a threat to the homeostasis of the body. He defines *stress* as the common systemic reactions to a stressor; bodily reactions that occur in response to exposure to threats. Such systemic reactions can be elicited by the wear and tear in the body caused by life, such as exposure to nervous tension, physical injury, infection, extreme heat or cold, and so on. According to Selye, stress responses are purposeful, homeostatic reactions, that is, the stress reactions serve as a protection to the body.[4] For example, let us consider the emotion *fear* caused by walking alone in the dark. Fear is a stressor that produces stress within the body. As a result of the stress, certain systemic reactions occur to protect the body, among which is a hypersecretion of cortisol and epinephrine which elevate the blood sugar and free fatty acids (FFA), thus providing for extra energy to flee from the dark, dilated pupils to permit better sight, and so on.

Disease is another stressor which elicits the systemic response in an effort to maintain a homeostatic equilibrium. If the disease is

[4] Hans Selye. The Stress of Life, Revised Edition, New York: McGraw-Hill Book Co., 1976, pp. 62, 78.

78

prolonged, or severe, the systemic response to it gradually weakens, and little "balancing" reserve remains to protect the body.

STRESSORS AND STRESSES OF EVERYDAY LIFE

Life would be short indeed, if the body could not withstand any threats or insults to it. Stressors and stress are normal constituents of life. A cold house on a wintry morning, a hot house on a summer day, a sleepless night, a sprained ankle, hunger, fear in the dark, a telegram with happy or sad news, an examination, an unexpected noise—all are stressors which produce systemic stress reactions in the body. Although some stressors are harmful, many are harmless, and the body, by its resiliency, is able to rebound, thus maintaining a state of balance, or homeostasis—dynamic equilibrium.

Stress cannot be avoided. An absence of it implies death. Contrary to the belief of some, prolonged bedrest is a great stressor which results in marked losses of nitrogen and potassium, a decrease in blood volume, and vasomotor disturbances, to name a few.

It has been said that stress is not nearly so important as the way a person perceives and handles it. Those who permit even the smallest events to hurt them will use their stress energy faster than those who take things in their stride. In general, people are predisposed to stress-related illnesses by virtue of their attitude toward other people and life-circumstances. These people are subject to such stress diseases as asthma, rheumatoid arthritis, migraine headaches, high blood pressure, ulcerative colitis, and peptic ulcer. It is important to note that while people are subjected to entirely different kinds of stressors, they may all experience the same physiological effects.

Body reactions to everyday stressors can be compared to the shock-absorbers on a car; as the shock-absorbers prevent a bumpy ride, the body's ability to adapt prevents undue harm, thus keeping it in a state of homeostatic balance, or health. On a wintry morning the body adapts by automatically constricting its peripheral blood vessels, thereby conserving body heat by shunting the blood to the more important internal organs that need it most. On a hot day, to prevent overheating, the body adapts by automatically sweating and dilating the peripheral blood vessels, thus permitting the dissipation of excessive body heat to the atmosphere.

When exposed to prolonged, or greatly intensified stressors, the body's ability to adapt and thus protect itself, gradually diminishes.

It is at this time that disease gains the upper hand, and the body is no longer in a state of dynamic balance. Shock is such a condition.

Disease, then, which can no longer be compensated for by the body's adaptive mechanisms, represents increased stress, or distress; an imbalanced body state—a disequilibrium which implies improper functioning of any or all of the four types of body cells. Just as a rowboat will capsize if all of its passengers are placed at one end of the boat, severe shock or death will occur when the body can no longer compensate for the stressors placed upon it, unless proper nursing care and treatment are administered rapidly.

Aging, especially premature aging, is, in a sense, due to the constant and eventual exhausting stresses of life. If pregnant women are exposed to unusually severe stressors, their fetuses could develop anomalies and malformations. This phenomenon has been called the syndrome of transmission. In persons who have sustained severe burns and infections, the anterior pituitary-adrenal cortical systems can become inactivated by exhaustive overstimulation. In such cases, corticosteroid treatment is of value.

According to Selye, the most nonspecific breakdown of resistance is shock. In such cases, autopsy reveals a characteristic triad of adrenocortical enlargement, thymicolymphatic atrophy, and bleeding in the gastrointestinal tract. Shock, then, is a disease of adaptation.[5]

SOCIALLY INDUCED STRESS

According to Rabkin and Struening, "the notion of socially induced stress as a precipitating factor in chronic diseases is gaining acceptance among a wide spectrum of scientists."[6] Social stressors refer to personal life changes which may alter a person's social setting. Although the exposure to such stressors does not, in itself, cause disease, it may alter a person's resistance and susceptibility, thus serving as a precipitating factor.

In the presence of strong social support systems, social stressors have only minor effects on health.

OUR DEFENSE REACTIONS: FIGHT OR FLIGHT

Any aggressor constitutes a threat to our homeostasis. We defend ourselves against aggressors in one of two ways: (1) by fighting—advanc-

[5] Ibid., p. 273.
[6] Rabkin and Struening, op. cit., pp. 1013–1020.

ing and attacking the enemy, or (2) by flight—retreating from the enemy. One has just to look back on our own childhood to understand this. Child A hits child B. Child B can do one of two things: (1) he can hit back, or (2) he can run away. Whichever he chooses to do, the child's main objective is to protect himself. Our body tissues use the same defense technique, i.e., fight or flight. For example, when microbes invade our bodies, our antibodies attack them—the fight mechanism. On the other hand, the accidental touching of a hot stove initiates the flight mechanism—a reflex reaction which causes the muscles to pull the hand away from the stove. Like the child, the body tries to protect itself. Like the man without a job, who draws upon his savings for survival, the body, under stress, draws upon its compensatory (adaptive) reserves to fight the aggressor.

SEVERE STRESS (DISTRESS) AND SUDDEN DEATH

There is reason to suspect that hope, purpose, meaning, and direction in life produce and maintain wellness, even in the face of adversity and stress. On the other hand, demorilization by the events and conditions of daily life predisposes one to illness, and, possibly, to sudden death.

Before 1900, physicians attributed sudden death to intense grief, fear, rage, or triumph. Later, during the advent of the germ theory of disease, there were doubts about these "folklore" beliefs, and they were discarded. Presently, we are returning to the notion that grief, fear, rage, triumph, and so on *do* play roles in sudden deaths.

In 1942, Dr. Walter Cannon wrote a paper which discussed possible physiological mechanisms in "voodoo death."[7] In 1957, a psychologist, Curt Richter, described an experiment in which healthy wild rats quickly gave up struggling and died when placed in a helpless situation.[8]

A recent study was done to analyze the life circumstances of 275 people who had suddenly died. From this study, four main categories emerged. (1) One hundred and thirty-five deaths were connected with an exceptionally traumatic separation of a close human relationship, or to a significant anniversary of the loss of a loved one. (2) One hundred and three deaths involved situations of personal danger, strug-

[7] Walter Cannon. "Voo Doo Death," *American Anthropologist*, **44**, 1942.
[8] George Engel. "Emotional Stress and Sudden Death," *Psychology Today*, (Nov. 1977), 114–118.

gle, fights, quarrels, or attack. (3) Twenty-one deaths involved loss of status, self-esteem, or valued possessions, disappointments, failure, or humiliation. (4) Sixteen people died in sudden moments of triumph, public recognition, reunion, or a "happy ending" situation. These four categories boil down to one common denominator: the victims were confronted with circumstances which they could not *ignore*. The most frequent emotions before sudden death seem to be those of giving up, helplessness, and hopelessness.[9]

DISPIRITING AND INSPIRITING EVENTS

According to Jourard, "all is not well" signals are pain, depression, boredom, frustration, anxiety, or general malaise. Dispiriting events increase our vulnerability to the forces of illness and disintegration. Such events are feelings of unimportance, worthlessness, hopelessness, low self-esteem, isolation, and frustration. On the other hand, inspiriting events give a sense of identity, worth, hope, purpose in living, and they mobilize the forces of wellness. A powerful statement made by Jourard is, "There is reason to suspect that hope, purpose, meaning, and direction in life produce and maintain wellness, even in the face of stress."[10]

STRESS AND SUSCEPTIBILITY TO ILLNESS

According to Wolf and Goodell, there is a relationship between psychological stress and an increased susceptibility to diseases. In terms of their theory, "The stress accruing from a situation is based in large part on the way the affected subject perceives it; perception depends upon a multiplicity of factors, including the genetic makeup, basic individual needs and longings, early conditioning influences, and a host of life experiences and cultural pressures."[11]

ROLE-BEHAVIOR AND STRESS

Stress energy is consumed when behavior is suppressed. When people wear masks, dreading to be known, then *other* people become

[9] Ibid.
[10] Sidney M. Jourald. *The Transparent Self,* Princeton: Van Nostrand, 1964, pp. 79–90.
[11] S. Wolf and H. Goodell. *Diary Council Digest,* **42** (May–June 1971), 14. Chicago: National Dairy Council.

sources of threat and stress to them. When people are obliged to play the role of spouse, friend, teacher, student, nurse, doctor, and so on in a stereotyped way, while withholding their inner "human" selves from the sight of others, it will follow that other people will never really come to know them. Not being known may be a relief, but it has its price.

SELYE'S PHILOSOPHY TO MINIMIZE STRESS AND DISTRESS

In his book, *Stress Without Distress,* Dr. Selye proposes a philosophical way of life which would decrease stress and distress by contributing toward man's happiness and satisfaction. He refers to this as "Altruistic Egotism," and emphasizes that while pure egotism leads to conflict and insecurity, the principle of Altruistic Egotism implies that all living beings are brothers; in the same boat, so to speak, and they are surprisingly *alike!* Earning the love of our fellow men should be our prime goal in life, and would help us to achieve peace and happiness. In so doing, unnecessary stresses of conflict, frustration, and hate could be avoided; hence, stress and distress could be minimized.[12]

STRESS AND GASTROINTESTINAL DISEASES

Of all the body systems, the gastrointestinal tract is especially vulnerable to stress.

The stomach

In animal studies, it was found that in threatening situations, motor activity and hydrochloric acid secretion in the stomach are brought to a halt. Although fright, depression, and feelings of being overwhelmed cause hypofunctioning of the stomach, aggressive attitudes, anger, resentment and frustration cause hyperfunctioning. Accompanying this are hyperemia and engorgement of the gastric mucosa, which leads to fragility of the gastric membranes, which in turn leads to small erosions and bleeding points. Hypersecretion of cortisol contributes to the weakness of the gastric mucosa through its gluconeogenesis action.* Increased sympathetic nervous system stimulation leads to vasoconstriction of gastrointestinal blood vessels, through the action

[12] Hans Selye. *Stress Without Distress,* New York: New American Library, 1974, p. 5.
* The breakdown of protein tissue resulting in an increased formation of glucose with a subsequent rise in liver glycogen and blood sugar.

of norepinephrine, thus decreasing the supply of substances to these cells. Cell weakness results.

The small intestine

Emotional stress leads to increased contraction of the duodenum, causing duodenal spasms. This can lead to obstruction of the biliary or pancreatic ducts causing biliary colic or acute pancreatitis.

The colon

Hostility leads to hyperfunctioning of the colon, hyperemic and fragile mucous membranes, and small bleeding points.

Mild depression and grim persistence cause constipation. On the other hand, fright or conflict, involving hostility, can result in watery diarrhea. In ulcerative colitis, diarrhea is almost continuous, with the hyperfunctioning, hyperemic colon with fragile mucous membranes leading to small bleeding points.

Hypotonia of the colon is characteristic of megacolon and postoperative ileus. This is frequently found in depressed persons.

STRESS AND CARDIOVASCULAR DISEASES

It is interesting to note that where there is civic pride and community cohesiveness, reverence for the elderly who remain useful, paternal heads of households—in a word, where there is mutual support and understanding, there is a low prevalence of cardiovascular diseases.

STRESS DISEASES AND CULTURAL DIFFERENCES

It seems quite probable that certain stress diseases are indigenous to different cultures. For example:

Europe and North America—Stress diseases are lung tumors from smoking, and cirrhosis from drinking.

Eastern Mediterranean—Malnutrition.

Japan and U.S. blacks—Essential hypertension. Not frequent in the blacks of Central and West Africa. Hypertension is unknown in New Guinea.

Widows and Divorcees—Increased incidence of peptic ulcers and tuberculosis.

Survivors of Wartime Concentration Camps—It is interesting to note that peptic ulcers were rare, along with a rarity of migraine, hyperthyroidism, appendicitis, gallstones, coronary heart disease and hypertension.[13]

In a study done in London by Wilson-Barnett and Carrigy, it was found that patients who were most vulnerable to stress and strong anxiety were

1. Those prone to high levels of anxiety and depression.
2. Females under 40 years of age.
3. Those who were hospitalized for the first time.
4. Those who were admitted for special tests.
5. Those with an undiagnosed illness, neoplastic disease, or infectious process.[14]

Explanations of procedures and hospital facilities, and preoperative patient-teaching, it was found, helped considerably to reduce patients' stress.[15]

The General Adaptation Syndrome (G.A.S.)

"The theory of the General Adaptation Syndrome is the most recent conceptual scheme devised to embrace all the various mechanisms through which the body responds to the 'stress of life.' "[16]

Throughout the centuries, a few great physiologists have searched for a common denominator relevent to all disease conditions. Among these are Claude Bernard, Walter B. Cannon, and Hans Selye.

In 1926, Dr. Selye first became aware that patients suffering from the most diverse diseases had a common look of illness as well as similar signs and symptoms, such as loss of appetite, decreased muscular strength, and loss of ambition. Many times there was a loss of weight. On their faces was a common look of illness. He also became aware that the same physiological alterations occurred in the bodies of animals subjected to different types of stressors, namely, enlargement of the

---

[13] "Society, Stress, and Disease," *World Health Organization Chronicle,* 2 (April 1971), 168–179.
[14] J. Wilson-Barnett and A. Carrigy. "Factors Influencing Patients' Emotional Reactions to Hospitalization," *Journal of Advanced Nursing* 3 (May 1978), 221–229. Oxford: Blackwell Scientific Publications. It would be interesting to determine the patient-categories of highest stress in the U.S.
[15] Ibid.
[16] René Dubos. Mirage of Health, New York: Harper and Row, 1959, pp. 100–101.

adrenal cortex, gastrointestinal ulcers, and involution of thymus and lymph nodes.

Dr. Selye hypothesized, and later proved experimentally, that every injury and disease causes two overall physiological reactions: (1) a local, or specific reaction involving a local part of the body, which he refers to as the Local Adaptation Syndrome, or L.A.S.,* and (2) a general, or nonspecific reaction involving the *whole* body, which he calls the General Adaptation Syndrome, or the G.A.S. (as it is universally abbreviated). The relationship between the L.A.S. and the G.A.S. is very close.

To quote Dr. Selye:

> It is as though we had hidden reserves of adaptability, or *adaptation energy,* in ourselves throughout the body. As soon as local stress consumes the most readily accessible local reserves, local exhaustion sets in and activity in the strained part stops automatically. This is an important protective mechanism, because, during the period of rest thus enforced, more adaptation energy can be made available, either from less readily accessible local stores or from reserves in other parts of the body. Only when all of our adaptability is used up will irreversible general exhaustion, and death ensue.[17]

According to Selye, our adaptation energies are finite; when we have exhausted our stores we die.

Let us consider an infected finger. The local, or specific reaction, involves the finger, per se, while the general, or nonspecific reaction involves the whole body as it mobilizes its forces to fight the infectious process. Or, we might compare the local adaptation syndrome and the general adaptation syndrome to the defense of a city. If the local city police (L.A.S.) are unable to quell a riot, the state police (G.A.S.) are called upon to assist. And so it is within the body; if the local stress becomes too severe, the G.A.S. is called into action to help defend the body, in an effort to maintain a state of health, or to help restore a state of health. The bedside care, the treatments, and the medications we administer are for the sole purpose of augmenting the body's defensive forces, and abating the aggressive threats to the patient's body.

---

* The L.A.S. elicits the inflammatory reaction: heat, swelling, redness, and pain which are always the same, and can be caused by a wide variety of agents, such as microorganisms, dust, x-ray, insect bites, plant pollens, and so on.
[17] Selye, *The Stress of Life,* Revised Edition, op. cit., p. 307.

STAGES OF THE GENERAL ADAPTATION SYNDROME

The general adaptation syndrome represents all nonspecific changes as they develop in the body throughout continued exposure to a stressor. The three stages of the G.A.S. are

The alarm reaction
The stage of resistance
The stage of exhaustion

The alarm reaction

No living organism can be maintained continuously in a state of alarm. The alarm reaction is the initial response to stress. Selye named it "alarm reaction" because he believed the syndrome probably represented the bodily expression of a generalized call-to-arms of the body's defensive forces. If the stressor is so damaging, or so profound that continuous exposure to it is incompatible with life, then death will ensue relatively rapidly. Otherwise, the alarm reaction will be followed by the second stage, the stage of resistance.

The stage of resistance

In this stage, the body resists the attack of the stressor. At this time, the body mobilizes its forces to fight the aggressor and to help maintain its status quo. The length of this stage is variable, as it is determined by the age, the general health (resistance) of the individual, and the nature and intensity of the stressor. When the individual is no longer able to resist the foe, the third and final stage of exhaustion follows.

The stage of exhaustion

This stage represents the period when the body can no longer compensate for the threats placed upon it; thus the body, unable to overthrow the aggressor, is in a state of marked disequilibrium.

If the stressor is not removed, there will be an eventual decline of the body's resistance, and an inevitable transition into the stage of exhaustion, at which time the body is no longer able to fight off its enemy. Unless prompt and proper medical and nursing management is instituted, death will follow this stage.

Although the entire general adaptation syndrome consists of the triad of stages, our efforts should be to prevent the third stage—the stage of exhaustion—or, if that is not possible, we should recognize the presence of the third stage and take vital steps to reverse the course.

Other principles applicable to the preceding are

PRINCIPLE 27:   Adaptation implies protection and survival.

PRINCIPLE 28:   The extent and course of an illness are the result of the degree to which the organism fails to adapt.

PRINCIPLE 29:   Failure to adapt results in disease or death.

If the stress is severe, the stage of exhaustion will occur rapidly; death can follow.

From what Selye has proposed and proved, i.e, that *all* emotional and physical illnesses are accompanied by a general, overall bodily response (the G.A.S.), it behooves us to understand the physiological mechanisms involved in this general response. When we have grasped the concept that the *whole* body is engaged to help the sick part, we will understand more fully the meaning of the worthiest of goals: to nurse the *whole* patient, instead of a part of the patient.

The Neuroendocrine Defenses of the Body

The nervous and endocrine systems are the two great coordinators of the general adaptation syndrome.

Before proceeding with the discussion of the neuroendocrine responses to stress, let us consider an analogy. By comparing the following chain of events to the neuroendocrine defense reactions, the reader might gain a better understanding of the functions of these two important coordinating systems, crucial in the defense of our bodies.

The President received authentic word that his country was in jeopardy. At once, he contacted the general to alert him that the country was in grave danger of attack. The general immediately issued orders to his colonels and majors to alert the military bases to prepare for action. The colonels and majors notified their respective bases and issued orders to the captains to release their troops at once to defend the country.

The lieutenants, along with their troops, were released, each troop having been trained to do a particular task requiring particular skills. At once they went to work to defend their country.

The different troops began their individual tasks, and, since they were stronger and more skilled, and far outnumbered the enemy, the enemy was conquered. Thus, the safety of the country was maintained. This story could have ended in another way, however.

Numerous strong troops were issued to fight an enemy as numerous and equally strong. The battle lasted for a long time, until finally, with prolonged and general exhaustion, together with a great loss of soldiers on both sides, the outcome hung in the balance. At last, one side waged a single, concerted final attack, and the war was over. Who won? Either side could have been victorious. Or, even another ending is possible.

The military bases, upon receipt of the orders, were compelled to send a few weak troops into the field to fight a strong enemy which far outnumbered them. The troops had been on constant duty defending their country against many small upsurges. Besides being weak, physically, they had suffered a gradual loss of soldiers. The results were fairly obvious; the enemy had the upper hand, so they won the war and took control of the country. Keep these analogies in mind as we proceed.

It has been pointed out that (1) the reaction to injury or disease is a phenomenon that involves the whole organism, and (2) every illness produces certain nonspecific effects on the body as a whole, including disturbances in organs and systems far removed from the injured area. The reaction to injury is known as the stress syndrome, of which the main regulators are the brain, nerves, pituitary gland, thyroid gland, adrenal glands, liver, kidneys, blood vessels, connective tissue cells, and white blood cells. The prevailing theory is that the systemic response to stress is initiated, coordinated, and sustained for a period of time by nervous and endocrine factors. We shall refer to these as defense mechanisms, compensatory mechanisms, or adaptive mechanisms.

Following severe bodily insult, such as occurs in shock, the "alarm reaction" is elicited, and the sympathetic nervous system is alerted to mobilize for "fight" or "flight" in order to defend the body. The nerve endings of the sympathetic nerves are stimulated to produce a chemical, norepinephrine, which causes vasoconstriction of most of the arterial and venous blood vessels of the body, especially those of the abdominal viscera and the skin of the extremities. (see Fig. 13.) Stimulated by the sympathetic nervous system directly, the heart rate and force are increased; hence, there is an increased output of blood from the heart into the aorta to the systemic circulation, and through the pulmonary artery to the pulmonary circulation. With the increased force and rate of the heart and the increased arteriolar resistance (resulting from the vasoconstrictor effects of norepinephrine), there is an increased venous return of blood to the heart; hence, an increased cardiac output, and systolic blood pressure.

The cerebral arteries of the brain and the coronary arteries to the myocardium are largely independent of sympathetic vasoconstrictor control. Blood flow through cerebral arteries is maintained at a level adequate to prevent brain damage, even at very low blood pressures. The coronary blood flow tends to decrease less than the myocardial work.

Although the vital body mechanisms are instantly mobilized to peak efficiency, the functioning of less vital parts decreases to a minimum level, which is evidence of an intelligent body economy. The objectives of this defense are (1) to maintain circulatory homeostasis, and (2) to provide for a depot of quick energy. It must always be remembered that an adequate supply of blood to the vital organs is necessary to sustain life. Blood is the only medium through which oxygen, nutrients, water, electrolytes, and hormones are supplied to these organs. Although less important parts of the body, such as the skin, also depend on a supply of blood, they can be deprived of it over a longer period of time with less untoward consequences.

THE ADRENAL MEDULLAE RESPONSES TO STRESS

There are two adrenal glands, each sits astride a kidney. The adrenal glands consist of an outer bark-like portion called the cortex, and an inner portion called the medulla. Of interest, however, is the fact that the cortex and the medulla are under different control—like a city within a city, each is governed independently of the other. Both adrenal cortical and adrenal medullary hormones play important roles in stress conditions; the adrenal medullary hormones play a greater role during acute emergencies than the cortical hormones.

The adrenal medulla is under the control of the sympathetic nervous system. Through the stimulation of the sympathetic nerve fibers innervating it, large quantities of epinephrine and norepinephrine are released from the adrenal medulla into the circulating blood stream which, in turn, transports them to various parts of the body. Approximately 75 per cent of the adrenal medullary secretion is norepinephrine, and 25 per cent is epinephrine. Under different physiological conditions, however, these relative proportions change considerably.

The adrenomedullary response is prompt, but it lasts only from one to twelve hours. Each of the adrenal medullary hormones will be considered separately.

Norepinephrine (an alpha receptor stimulator)

Norepinephrine is identical to Cannon's sympathin E; "E" meaning *excitor mechanism.* Trade names for norepinephrine are Levophed, Noradrenalin, and so on.

The adrenal medullary output of norepinephrine augments that produced by the sympathetic nervous system. The chief value of norepinephrine lies in its potent vasoconstrictor effect on arterial blood vessels through its action on the alpha receptors of the smooth muscle layer of these vessels. The result of this is an increased arterial blood pressure. Another value of norepinephrine is its constricting effect on the veins. Initially, increased venous constriction results in an increased venous return of blood to the right atrium. Since the left side of the heart can only pump out into the arterial circuit the amount of blood it receives from the right side of the heart, this is a beneficial adjunct to cardiac output. Norepinephrine also causes increased activity of the heart, inhibition of the gastrointestinal tract, and dilation of the pupils of the eyes.

Epinephrine (a beta receptor stimulator)

The trade name for epinephrine is Adrenalin. Epinephrine is believed to be produced especially during emergencies, such as emotional crises, hypoglycemia, mild hypoxia, and hypotension—all of which are stress conditions. Three fourths of its action is through beta receptors, and about one fourth of its action is on alpha receptors.

The effects of epinephrine on the body are as follows:

1. Through its action on the beta receptors of the heart, epinephrine increases the rate and force of the heart beat, thereby increasing the cardiac output and increasing the systolic blood pressure. Large amounts of epinephrine (or Adrenalin administered over a prolonged period of time) can be detrimental to cardiac performance. A very rapid heart rate decreases cardiac filling time, myocardial efficiency, cardiac output, and coronary blood flow. It can also cause cardiac arrhythmias, including fibrillation. A prolonged curtailment of blood flow can lead to an intense stagnant anoxia in visceral organs, from

which sites acid and/or toxic factors can be released into the circulation. As a consequence, metabolic acidosis becomes increasingly dangerous, and the toxic factors may exert harmful effects on the cardiovascular system.

Propranolol HCL (Inderal), a beta adrenergic blocking drug, is frequently administered to block the effects of epinephrine on the heart, and to restore a more normal rhythm. And so it can be seen that while a little bit of epinephrine is good, too much can lead to dangerous effects—as is evident with all of nature.

2. Epinephrine dilates the bronchioles of the lungs by relaxing the smooth muscle, thereby aiding the gaseous exchange of oxygen and carbon dioxide (an important treatment in asthma and anaphylactic shock).

3. Epinephrine dilates the coronary blood vessels of the heart and of the blood vessels of the muscles.

4. Epinephrine exerts minor constrictor effects on the blood vessels of the skin (with minor stimulation of alpha receptors), and on kidneys, with a subsequent shunt of blood from the constricted areas to the dilated areas. Ordinary amounts of epinephrine lessen peripheral resistance, while larger than physiologic doses causes predominant constrictor effects.

5. Epinephrine increases the metabolic rate often as much as 150 per cent above normal, thereby increasing the activity and excitability of the whole body. It also increases the total oxygen consumption by up to 30 per cent. This calorigenic action is due largely to the metabolism of lactate in the liver, and also to increased work of the heart and muscles of respiration.

6. Epinephrine raises the blood sugar (hyperglycemia) by increasing the breakdown of glycogen in the liver (glycogenolysis), thereby causing it to release more glucose into the blood stream. Although the rate of insulin-release is not proportionate to the amount of epinephrine, the tissues do not receive the benefit of the additional glucose as much as the brain benefits by it (the metabolism of glucose in the brain is not dependent upon insulin). The increased hyperglycemia is sometimes to levels high enough to produce glucosuria.

7. Epinephrine increases sweating, thus causing the dissipation of excessive body heat.

8. Epinephrine decreases gastrointestinal peristalsis.

9. Epinephrine dilates the pupils of the eyes.

10. Epinephrine hastens the clotting process when injected into the body. Emotional excitement, muscular exercise, and hemorrhage act similarly, probably through the liberation of epinephrine from the adrenal medullae. Epinephrine has no effect on the coagulation of blood after it has been shed.

11. There is considerable evidence that excitation of the adrenal medullae causes contraction of the spleen which, consequently, squeezes blood into the general circulation. In stress due to blood loss, this affords compensatory assistance by increasing the blood volume.

12. Epinephrine increases the formation of blood lactate, as the result of rapid glycogenolysis in skeletal muscle. The lactate is carried to the liver where it is converted to glycogen, and to the heart where it provides energy for contraction.

13. Epinephrine releases free fatty acids (FFA) from adipose tissue, which can be used to provide energy. FFA is elicited by exercise and emotional stimuli, i.e., anger, depression, and fear. A study done by Cobb et al. revealed that hypnotized subjects had increased levels of FFAs when they relived emotional experience and exercise by hypnotic suggestion.[18]

14. Epinephrine, to a minimum extent, stimulates the production of ACTH which, in turn, stimulates the production of adrenal cortical hormones.

15. Epinephrine may inhibit the release of the antidiuretic hormone (ADH) from the posterior pituitary gland.

16. Epinephrine is used clinically for the following:
Anaphylactic shock
Treatment of bronchial asthma
Urticaria
Cardiac failure

17. In combination with local anesthetics in eye, nose, and throat surgery, as well as superficial skin suturing, epinephrine constricts superficial blood vessels and decreases bleeding.

18. In the treatment of insulin shock, epinephrine causes a rapid release of glucose from the liver, thus raising the blood sugar.

[18] L. A. Cobb, H. S. Ripley and J. W. Jones. "Free Fatty Acid Mobilization During Suggestion of Exercise and Stress Using Hypnosis and Sodium Amytol," *Psychosomatic Medicine* **35** (Sept.–Oct. 1973), 367–374.

19. The catecholamines (epinephrine and norepinephrine) directly increase the release of renin from the juxtaglomerular cells which adjoin the glomeruli of the kidneys. Renin, in turn, stimulates the production of angiotensin which is a powerful stimulator of peripheral blood vessels, causing them to constrict. Too, angiotensin stimulates the adrenal cortex to secrete copious amounts of aldosterone which, in turn, conserves sodium and water. These two mechanisms, i.e., vasoconstriction and fluid-retention assist in elevating the blood pressure in emergency situations. In hypertensive subjects, however, this could be lethal.

20. Epinephrine and norepinephrine cause the erection of hair, or goose flesh, due to the contraction of the arrectores pili muscles.

ADVERSE EFFECTS OF THE USE OF ADRENALIN

Tremors, dyspnea, chills, increased apprehension, nausea, vomiting, cyanosis, perspiration, and headache may result from the administration of Adrenalin. In any kind of hypovolemic shock, in which the myocardium is ischemic, adrenalin is a dangerous drug to use, because it could cause death by ventricular fibrillation. Since one of the actions of adrenalin is to increase cardiac irritability, this action is enhanced if myocardial blood flow is decreased.

To sum up: the adrenal medulae, under the control of the sympathetic nervous system, release two hormones (catecholamines or adrenergics) which initiate very similar effects to those caused by direct sympathetic stimulation, i.e., increased heart rate and vasoconstriction. The only significant differences are caused by the epinephrine, which increases body metabolism and cardiac output to a greater degree than does the sympathetic nervous system. While the adrenal medullary secretion is not necessary to maintain life, it is, however, an adjunct to the adrenal cortex in aiding the body to cope with acute stress.

Both epinephrine and norepinephrine, in times of severe stress such as shock, initiate the catabolism of fatty tissue (lipolysis). It has been demonstrated experimentally that these two catecholamines accelerate the catabolism of triglycerides to free fatty acids (FFA) and glycerol. Glucocorticoids and thyroid hormones also increase fat metabolism. While this increased fat metabolism is beneficial for use as fuel in producing energy (ATP), there is an inherent danger of metabolic acidosis because of the large quantities of ketone bodies formed. The liver, unfortunately, cannot keep pace in oxidizing them.

ALPHA AND BETA RECEPTORS

At various sites within the smooth muscle of the circulatory system (arteries and veins), are alpha and beta receptor sites which respond to the catecholamines epinephrine and norepinephrine by either vasoconstriction or vasodilatation. Beta receptors are also located in the heart muscle.

Alpha receptors

When stimulated, alpha receptors, located primarily in the peripheral arterioles and veins, respond by constricting these vessels. The chief catecholamine which stimulates these receptors is norepinephrine. Although norepinephrine can also stimulate beta receptors, it does so to a much lesser degree than epinephrine. To reiterate, the main function of norepinephrine is to stimulate alpha receptors of the blood vessels to cause vasoconstriction.

Beta receptors

Beta receptor sites (like the alphas) are also located in the peripheral arteries and veins, in the arteries of the heart, skeletal muscles, and bronchioles of the lungs. When stimulated, primarily by epinephrine, the heart contracts more rapidly (chronotropic effect) and forcefully (inotropic effect), the arteries of the heart and periphery dilate, and the bronchioles dilate. Epinephrine exerts both alpha and beta responses equally, and it is more potent than norepinephrine as a vasoconstrictor agent. However, according to Best and Taylor, norepinephrine may produce a greater vasoconstriction and elevation of blood pressure because it does not have any effect on the beta receptors (dilating receptors) as does epinephrine.[19] This may appear confusing; another way to say it is: while epinephrine is a greater vasoconstrictor than is norepinephrine, this is offset somewhat by its ability to act on beta receptors, too, thus somewhat neutralizing the effects of vasoconstriction.

It was formerly thought that alpha receptors played no role on

[19] *Best and Taylor's Physiological Basis of Medical Practice,* 9th Ed., John R. Brobeck (ed.), Baltimore: Williams and Wilkins Co., 1973, pp. 9–64.

Drug	Stimulatory Action	Effector Site	Clinical Indication
Epinephrine (Adrenalin)	Beta and Alpha (equally)	Increased heart rate (chronotrophic) Increased force of myocardial con- tractions (ino- trophic) Increased velocity of A-V conduc- tion	Cardiovascular collapse Bradycardia Adam's-Stokes attacks Bronchial asthma
Norepinephrine (Levophed)	Alpha, primarily	Increased peripheral vascular resistance. Increased BP.	Cardiovascular shock
Isoproterenol (Isuprel)	Beta	Similar to epin- ephrine	Bradycardia, with or without heart block
Metaraminol (Aramine)	Alpha	Similar to norepin- ephrine	Cardiovascular collapse and cardiogenic shock
Methoxamine (Vasoxyl)	Alpha	Similar to norepin- ephrine	Cardiogenic shock
Phenyephrine (Neosynephrine)	Alpha	Similar to norepin- ephrine	Cardiogenic shock
Mephentermine (Wyamine)	Beta, primarily	Similar to epin- ephrine	Cardiovascular collapse

Figure 12. *Alpha and beta drugs.*

the heart, however, a recent study by Rabine et al. suggests the presence of alpha and beta adrenergic receptors in the human atrium.[20]
They conclude that epinephrine can induce both slowing and acceleration of the spontaneous rate of atrial fibers.

ALPHA AND BETA DRUGS

Some drugs are alpha stimulators, causing vasoconstriction of peripheral blood vessels; some are beta stimulators, causing peripheral

[20] L. M. Rabine, A. J. Hordof, F. O. Bowman, J. R. Malm and M. R. Rosen. "Alpha
and Beta Andrenergic Effects on Human Atrial Specialized Conducting Fibers," *Circulation* **57** (Jan. 1978), 88.

vasodilatation, bronchial dilatation, and inotrophic and chronotrophic effects on the heart. Some drugs exert both alpha and beta actions. (See Fig. 12.)

Alpha blocking drugs

Some drugs block the effects of alpha adrenergic catecholamines:

1. Reserpine prevents the synthesis and storage of norepinephrine in the sympathetic nerve endings.
2. Guanethidine blocks the release of norepinephrine from the sympathetic nerve endings.
3. Phenoxybenzamine and phentolamine (Regitine) block the alpha receptors. Sympathetic activity can be blocked by drugs which block the transmission of sympathetic and parasympathetic nerve impulses through the autonomic ganglia. An example of such a drug is hexamethonium.

Beta blocking drugs

Propranolol (Inderal) blocks the beta receptors. Beta blockers cause mild vasoconstriction and they inhibit the positive inotrophic and chronotrophic effects of catecholamines and sympathetic stimulation of the heart. A beta blocker is a very useful drug, as, at times, increased amounts of catecholamines and increased sympathetic stimulation lead to cardiac arrhythmias. Beta blockers act on the sinoatrial node to decrease the spontaneous heart rate, and on the atrioventricular conduction system to slow the rate with which stimuli are transmitted to the ventricle from the atrium. Since increased stimulation of the beta receptors in the heart causes cardioacceleration, this can be detrimental to cardiac performance. A very rapid heart rate decreases cardiac filling time, myocardial efficiency, cardiac output, and coronary blood flow. It can also cause cardiac arrhythmias, including fibrillation.

The Sympathetic Nervous System and Adrenal Medullary Defenses in Action

The sympathoadrenal medullary response, we said, is an automatic preparation for emergency situations, such as for fight or flight. For example, let us say that you worked late one night. You got off the bus and had three long blocks to walk along a dark street before reaching home. You were weary, and the thought of walking the three long blocks didn't help any. All of a sudden, as if out of nowhere, you felt a heavy hand on your shoulder! What was your reaction? It could have been one of two reactions: You could have stayed and fought, or you could have run away—the fight or flight mechanism.

You decided to run away. You had two and a half blocks to go. Let us trace how your sympathoadrenal medullary responses helped you to get home. The heavy hand on your shoulder was the stressor that initiated the alarm reaction in your body to mobilize your compensatory forces. The compensatory forces, in turn, would help you to cope with this stress situation. Your liver poured out excessive amounts of glucose into your blood stream to give you quick energy. In turn, this glucose was carried rapidly via a faster-moving blood stream to your leg muscles, whose blood vessels were dilated to receive it. You could feel your heart pounding rapidly; its rate was accelerated in order to provide your leg muscles with additional quantities of blood. Your constricted skin vessels also provided your leg muscles with more

Figure 13. *The sympathetic-adrenal medullary responses to stressors.*

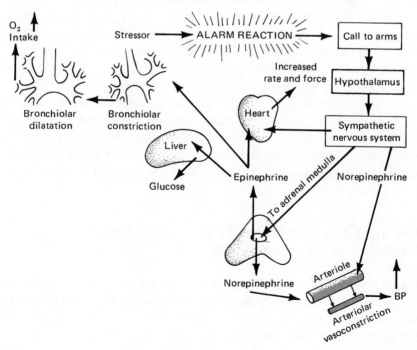

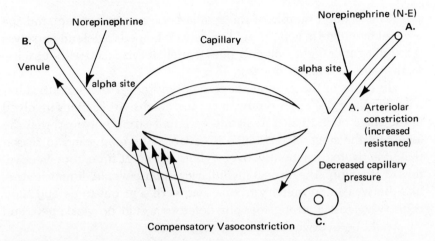

Figure 14. *Compensatory Vasoconstriction.*
   A. Action of norepinephrine on the arteriole: arteriolar vasoconstriction leads to decreased capillary pressure. The colloid osmotic pressure is thus enhanced at the venous end of the capillary, and large amounts of fluid leave the interstitial compartment and enter the vascular compartment.
   B. Norepinephrine also causes venous constriction. Initially, in shock, large volumes of blood are squeezed from the veins to the right atrium. Continuous venous constriction leads to increased capillary pressure; and fluids will be forced back into the interstitial compartment.
   C. There is a marked decrease of the five substances to the cells. If the vasoconstriction is prolonged, metabolic acidosis will occur.

blood, as the blood was shunted from the constricted vessels to the dilated ones. Your dilated bronchioles permitted you to inhale additional amounts of fresh air, and to exhale large amounts of carbon dioxide accumulating in your body as the result of increased muscular exercise. The pupils of your eyes dilated, thus permitting you to see your way better.

You finally reached home! Locking the door behind you, you leaned back against it and trembled. Glancing into a mirror opposite the door, you noticed how pale you looked, and your skin was covered with perspiration. Although you felt very warm, your skin felt cold.

The flight was over. You marveled at the extra spurt of energy. "Where did it come from?" you thought. "When I got off the bus, I was almost too tired to put one foot in front of the other." And you never knew you could run so fast.

This is one example of the sympathetic nervous system and the adrenal medullae in action, and how we are helped to defend ourselves through fight or flight. Not only does fear elicit this reaction, but excitement, rage, and anger do also.

In terms of the general adaptation syndrome, the sympathoadrenal medullary responses typify one of the defensive reactions involved in the stage of resistance. It should be emphasized, however, that the length of the stage of resistance is variable. It would stand to reason that, if activated frequently, over a short period of time, the effectiveness of the sympathoadrenal medullary response would diminish. And, like the weakened military troops that were sent out to defend their country against a strong foe, our defenses would be weakened, and we would be overwhelmed by our aggressor.

ADRENAL CORTICAL RESPONSES TO STRESS

Of the two systemic responses to stress, the nervous and the endocrine, the endocrine is the latest to be discovered. An adequate endocrine response is necessary for survival, i.e., an adequate response is necessary for the body's successful resistance to harmful stimuli. This does not mean that the most intense response is necessarily the most beneficial. An excessive response to the alarm reaction may even be detrimental.

The hormonal response to stress results in the provision of emergency fuel such as amino acids, fatty acids, glucose, sodium, and water for the cells, tissues, organs, and systems. To make its fuel, the body breaks down food into amino acids, fatty acids, and glucose. Then, in order to turn these into energy, a chemical process occurs in the body that results in the formation of adenosine triphosphate (ATP). ATP is the main source of energy made and used inside the cells. In his discussion on shock, Selye stated that

> Increased corticoid production is one of the fundamental steps in the defense against systemic stress, and the corticoids, in turn, play an important role in gluconeogenesis from protein, the utilization of sugar, and protein-degradation products, as well as the metabolism of sodium.[21]

It has been proved that a constant level of adrenalcortical hormones provides for survival over a wide range of stressful situations: physical, psychological, and emotional. Let us dissect these hormonal

[21] Selye, *The Stress of Life*, Revised Ed., op. cit., p. 106.

mechanisms to see what unique features they possess in providing for survival.

THE ANTERIOR PITUITARY GLAND

The anterior pituitary gland is the "master gland" of the body; it stands first in importance of all the glands that produce hormones. This master gland is about the size of a pea, and is suspended just below the center of the brain. Because of its location, it is thought to be under direct control of the hypothalamus of the brain, however, no distinct nerve connections between the two have been established. We do know, however, that hypothalamic control of the anterior pituitary gland exists, as any damage to the hypothalamus affects the anterior pituitary gland also.

THE TROPIC HORMONES OF THE ANTERIOR PITUITARY GLAND

The anterior pituitary gland produces tropic hormones that control growth, sexual development, reproduction, thyroid activity, and, to an important extent, the body's general response to stress. This control, in most instances, is a two-stage process; tropic hormones from the anterior pituitary gland regulate the hormonal secretion of its target endocrine glands, such as the adrenal cortex, thyroid gland, thymus gland, ovaries, and testes. Of the seven tropic hormones produced by the anterior pituitary, the most important during stress are considered to be the growth hormone and the adrenocorticotropic hormone (ACTH). For the purposes of this book, only ACTH, which stimulates the adrenal cortex, will be discussed. Figure 15 is a diagrammatic illustration of the effects of ACTH on the adrenal cortex. Understanding might be facilitated if this figure is referred to while reading the following.

The adrenocorticotropic hormone (ACTH, corticotropin)

ACTH, secreted by the anterior pituitary, stimulates the adrenal cortex to produce three groups of adrenal cortical hormones which are classified as (1) mineralocorticoids, (2) glucocorticoids, and (3) weak androgens. Generally speaking, the mineralocorticoids control fluid and electrolyte balance, while the glucocorticoids affect energy and tissue resistance.

When the body is in stress, the anterior pituitary secretes ACTH in abundance which, in turn, stimulates the adrenal cortex to secrete

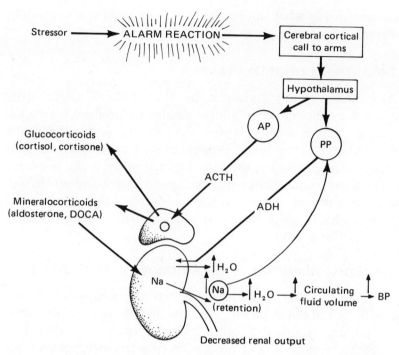

Figure 15. *The adrenal cortical and ADH responses to stressors. (ACTH) Adrenocorticotropic hormone, (ADH) antidiuretic hormone, (AP) anterior pituitary gland, (DOCA) desoxycorticosterone acetate, (PP) posterior pituitary gland.*

large amounts of its hormones into the general circulation. Of the various hormones released from the adrenal cortex, however, only cortisol (hydrocortisone) of the glucocorticoid group has a feedback inhibitory effect on the anterior pituitary gland. In other words, a high level of cortisol in the blood stream would cause a decrease in the secretion of ACTH by the anterior pituitary gland. In health, this check and balance system maintains the level of circulating plasma-cortisol within relatively narrow limits. If there is a stressful situation, however, the anterior pituitary gland increases its output of ACTH, irrespective of the level of circulating cortisol.

ADRENAL CORTICAL HORMONES

The adrenal corticoids (or corticosteroids) produce metabolic changes within the body which influence the behavior of water, sodium, carbohydrates, and protein. Shock due to adrenal cortical failure is, in part, due to hypoglycemia and to an electrolyte imbalance.

Glucocorticoids (cortisol and cortisone)

A wide variety of stressors can stimulate the secretion of glucocorticoids. A few of these stressors are trauma, intense heat or cold, surgical operations, physical restraint, and most debilitating diseases. A basic level of corticoids permits a satisfactory total metabolic response of the body over a relatively wide range of adverse conditions.

As the name "glucocorticoid" implies, one of the most important actions of these hormones is *gluconeogenesis,* the breakdown of protein tissue resulting in an increased formation of glucose with a subsequent rise in liver glycogen and blood sugar. Nerve cells cannot survive without glucose, therefore, gluconeogenesis is especially important during stress. Glucocorticoids make available the stored reserves of ready energy by rapidly mobilizing glycogen, fat, amino acids, and tissue protein from their cellular stores, thus making them available for energy. Glucocorticoids do not usually mobilize basic functional cellular proteins, such as contractile proteins of muscle fiber, until almost all other protein has been released. Glucocorticoids can also decrease inflammatory responses and reduce the severity of allergic reactions by preventing fibrosis, minimizing degeneration, decreasing capillary permeability at the injured site, and increasing phagocytosis of exudate. It is thought that these effects might be caused by the tendency of glucocorticoids to decrease the formation of cell proteins, such as immune bodies, that are responsible for allergic and inflammatory reactions. On the heart, glucocorticoids have inotrophic and chronotrophic effects.

Even though there is a great deal more to be learned about the effects of glucocorticoids, it has, nevertheless, been established that they play a very important role in sustaining life. A complete absence of glucocorticoids renders the body unable to cope with any form of physical or mental stress. Minor illnesses in such individuals could lead to death.

Mineralocorticoids

Mineralocorticoids are of fundamental importance in maintaining the fluid and electrolyte balance of the body by regulating the absorption and excretion of sodium, potassium, and water. Aldosterone and desoxycorticosterone (D.O.C.) belong to this group of hormones; of the two, aldosterone is the more important. Through its action on

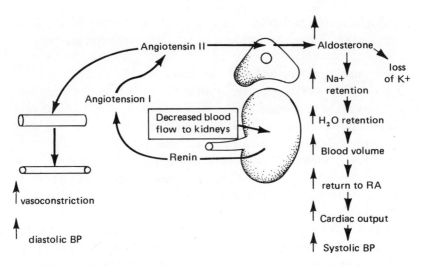

Figure 16. *Effects of renal ischemia.*

the renal tubules, aldosterone promotes the reabsorption of sodium (hence, water), chloride, and the elimination of potassium.

In a study done by Foster as a means of determining nursing effectiveness in reducing patients' stress, she found the trends in the sodium/potassium ratio to be an indicator of stress. The results of her study suggest that the urinary sodium/potassium ratio is a valid index for the body's biochemical response to stress, and thus reflective of patient-welfare.[22]

The production of aldosterone is controlled by several factors, among which are ACTH, decreased blood volume, dehydration, decreased body-sodium, increased potassium, the growth hormone (STH), and, perhaps the most potent stimulator of them all—angiotensin. (See Fig. 16.) Decreased blood pressure in the arterioles supplying the renal glomeruli leads to an increased secretion of renin by the kidney, which, in turn, increases angiotensin which leads to an acceleration in the secretion of aldosterone. In the section dealing with hypovolemia, we shall see the value of this hormone in action.

The posterior pituitary gland: antidiuretic hormone (ADH)

The antidiuretic hormone (ADH), secreted by the posterior pituitary gland, plays an important role in helping to maintain the homeo-

[22] Sue B. Foster. "An Adrenal Measure for Evaluating Nursing Effectiveness," *Nursing Research* 23 (March–April 1974), 118–124.

static equilibrium of the body. The osmolality of the blood affects the secretion of the ADH, i.e., the greater the concentration of sodium in the blood, the greater is the amount of secretion of antidiuretic hormone. The presence of ADH greatly accelerates the reabsorption of water in the body. Acute volume depletion following hemorrhage is one of the most potent stimuli for the release of ADH, even more than the response due to increased osmolality of the blood. In subsequent chapters, we shall see how this hormone is beneficial in conditions of shock.

THE THYROID GLAND

During stress, increased thyrotropic hormones (TSH) are produced and secreted into the blood stream for the purpose of increasing metabolism in every tissue of the body.

Indicators of stress (signs of danger)

Typical laboratory data

Blood:
↑ Epinephrine*
↑ Norepinephrine
↑ Glucocorticoids
↑ ACTH
↓ Eosinophiles
↑ Creatine/creatinine ratio
↑ Cholesterol
↑ FFA (free fatty acids)
↑ Blood Pressure

Self-observable signs

1. Irritability, hyperexcitable, depression, keyed up
2. Pounding of the heart
3. Dry mouth and throat
4. Impulsive and unstable, emotionally
5. Decreased ability to concentrate
6. Fatigue
7. Floating anxiety

* The ↑ sign means "increased"; ↓ means "decreased."

8. Nervous tics
9. Grinding of the teeth
10. Insomnia
11. Excessive sweating
12. Frequent need to urinate
13. Indigestion, diarrhea, anorexia
14. Headaches
15. Neck or low back pain
16. Nightmares
17. Accident-prone

It is hoped that by the time this book has been read, the reader will be able to figure out the altered physiological reasons for each of these.

REFERENCES

Anderson, Marcia D., and Jane M. Pleticha. "Emergency Unit Patients' Perceptions of Stressful Life Events." *Nursing Research,* **23** (Sept.–Oct. 1974), 378–383.

Kramer, Marlene, and Patricia Benner. "Role Conceptions and Integrative Role Behavior of Nurses in Special Care and Regular Hospital Nursing Units." *Nursing Research,* **21** (Jan.–Feb. 1972), 20–29.

Rahe, R. H., et al. "Social Stress and Illness Onset." *Journal Psychosomatic Res* (July 1964), 35–44.

Selye, Hans. "They All Looked Sick to Me." *Human Nature,* **1** (Feb. 1978), 58–63.

Toffler, Alvin. *Future Shock.* New York: Random House, 1970.

CHAPTER 7

Physiological-Psychological Aspects of the "Whole" Patient: Implications for the Nursing Profession

"Nothing can happen to the body which is not perceived by the mind."
—*Spinoza*

The "Whole" Patient

". . . man interacts as an integrated whole with the totality of the environment."
—*Martha E. Rogers*[1]

We must consider the cell in proper perspective with the tissue, the tissue in turn with the organ, the organ in turn with the organism. Final emphasis must be on the individual as a whole, rather than on a small bit of tissue—we are interested in a *total* system complex.[2]

That there is a general, overall physiological response of the body to emotional upsets, injury, and disease has been well established. Today, the concept of the General Adaptation Syndrome is widely accepted by major medical authorities who are applying it to their management of the "whole" patient. It is rare not to read something about "homeo-

[1] Martha E. Rogers. *An Introduction to the Theoretical Basis of Nursing*, Philadelphia: F. A. Davis Co., 1970, p. 50.
[2] Howard C. Hopps. *Principles of Pathology*, 2nd Ed., New York: Appleton-Century-Crofts, 1964, p. 13.

stasis," "stress," and the "General Adaptation Syndrome" in current medical journals of the world. The nursing profession, on the other hand, has not been as progressive in its thinking or practice. With good intentions, we conscientiously mouthe such pet phrases as: "We should nurse the *whole* patient, rather than just a part of the patient"; "*Total* nursing care"; "*Comprehensive* nursing care"; and "Holistic approach," yet somewhere along the line the true meaning of these words has eluded us. The key words in the previous statements are "whole," "total," "comprehensive," and "holistic"—and the ways we have interpreted these words have arrested our progress. It would behoove our profession to arrive at *one* common meaning!

Physical Versus Psychological and Emotional Aspects of Care

> Neither the psyche nor the soma should hold the limelight. They comprise but halves of the same circle, without beginning or end but with varying, alternating or even coincidental lengths of arc. We cannot well consider them separately. We must put the body together again. . . . —Paul Dudley White[3]

Implicit in every physical illness is an emotional reaction to that illness. Implicit in every emotional disturbance is a physiological response, or reaction, to that disturbance. Or, we might say that the psyche affects the soma, and the soma affects the psyche. There is really no separation of the two.

Like physiological reactions, emotional reactions often constitute unconscious mechanisms through which man attempts to defend himself against threats. For example, protective reaction patterns to stressful life situations are anger, resentment, hostility, anxiety, apprehension, passivity, and so on. Over a period of time, these can lead to ulceration and hemorrhage.

It is known that fright, depression, and feelings of being overwhelmed cause hypofunction (sympathetic nervous system mediation) of the gastrointestinal tract, while aggressive attitudes such as anger and resentment, cause hyperfunction (parasympathetic mediation).

According to Luborsky, et al., the most frequent physiological antecedents of somatic illness are resentment (hostility), frustration

[3] Paul Dudley White. "The Psyche and the Soma: The Spiritual and Physical Attributes of the Heart," *Annals of Internal Medicine,* 35 (Dec. 1951), 1291.

(rejection), depression (hopelessness), anxiety, helplessness, separation, and life change. Disorders such as migraine headache, duodenal ulcers, and asthma may occur during post-stress periods. They are illnesses which are fundamentally mediated through the parasympathetic nervous system.[4]

Up until about thirty years ago, the main emphasis of nursing and nurse educators was placed on the physical needs of patients. Then came the sudden and swift transition. The pendulum swung in the opposite direction, with the emphasis on the psychological-emotional needs of patients. Physical—psychological—emotional—did these not comprise the "whole"? mused our nursing educators. Assuming that it did, and realizing the earlier deemphasis of psychological and emotional needs, nursing leaders changed the curricula; more and more courses were incorporated in order to provide for a better understanding of the emotional and psychological aspects of the patient. The physiological alterations accompanying the psychological aspects were disregarded. In many instances, there were no changes made in the basic science aspects of the curricula. While all-out attempts were made to integrate and correlate aspects dealing with psychological and emotional needs, basic sciences took a back seat! Little effort was made to integrate and correlate science courses throughout the nursing curricula.

The results of these past decades have not proved to be especially strengthening to our profession. Medical and surgical patients desire and deserve, first and foremost, those services which will assist them to become physically well again, insofar as this is possible. In the majority of these instances, to "become well" necessitates that nurses have knowledge and understanding of the physiological processes involved, along with a firm understanding of the normal processes.

According to McLeod, "Although a majority of nurses work with physically ill persons, only a small proportion of currently reported nursing research is concerned with physical care, with normal or pathophysiology, or with the physiological need for or effects of nursing intervention."[5]

One nurse might spend hours trying to find out why a patient

[4] Docherty L. Luborsky and P. Sydnor. "Onset Conditions for Psychosomatic Symptoms: A Comparative Review of Immediate Observation with Retrospective Research," *Psychosomatic Medicine*, 35 (May–June 1973), 187–204.
[5] Dorothy L. McLeod. "Physiological Model," in *Theoretical Issues in Professional Nursing*, Juanita F. Murphy (Ed.), New York: Appleton-Century-Crofts, 1971, pp. 1, 14.

is disgruntled by talking to him. Another nurse might brush the crumbs from his bed, or give him a needed laxative, or rub his back, and see the disgruntled behavior disappear.

On the other side of the coin, for example, a patient's fears about his pending surgery cannot be alleviated through physical care; his emotional needs must be managed with patient-teaching—purposeful conversation. To nurse one aspect without due consideration and appreciation of the other could only result in ineffectual nursing care. Newman identified three major psychological needs of medical-surgical patients: (1) psychological needs derived from fear, anxiety, pain, and loneliness, (2) the psychological need to exercise control over himself, and (3) the psychological need to have his identity recognized and maintained during disability. She points out that number 1 is the most frequent need.[6]

Ironically, to give physical care is *also* to give emotional care. The majority of patients perceive physical care as being an emotional support *also*, as the nurse is doing something to or for him to aid his recovery; this tells him that she cares about him. She is one human being taking care of another human being to sustain his life. In that sense, psychological-emotional support is built into physical care. On the other hand, we all know the impersonal robot-type nurse who conveys the impression that the patient does not really exist; she regards him as a dehumanized "thing." The patient perceives her behavior as insulting, demoralizing, and dispiriting. If he is acutely ill, this could well be devastating to him, both psychologically and physiologically.

Then there is the oversolicitous nurse who, recognizing a patient's expression of fear or anxiety, moves in and talks with him, trying to unearth the reason for this seemingly emotional-psychological problem. She pulls up a chair (which is fine, if done at the proper time and in the proper context), grabs his hand, and engages in a lengthy discourse, during which, and all the while, the patient's fear and anxious expression may be due to a *physiological* deficit, such as decreased circulation of blood to the brain. Had she made a physiological assessment *before* she assumed that his anxiety was solely psychologically based, her nursing actions may have been quite different.

Perhaps one of the greatest challenges facing nurses today is to

[6] Kay Corman Kintzel. *Advanced Concepts in Nursing*, Philadelphia: J. B. Lippincott Co., 1971, p. 73.

gain the knowledge and the wisdom to judge, scientifically, the type of care that *should* be given to patients.

The nurse should not impose further insults on an ill patient whose body is already under stress and out of tune. She should be cognizant of her facial expressions, body movements, eye contact, and tone of her voice. Since all sensory input takes place through the five senses, the nurse should be aware that some of hers might be stressful to the patient.

Situations which greatly increase or decrease the sensory input could overtax an already exhausted patient. According to Kintzel, "Disturbances in environmental stimulation or sensory input may be classified into three operational processes: 1) sensory deprivation, 2) sensory overload, and 3) sensory distortion, in which an auditory stimulus, for example, is presented out of proper time sequence with tactile and visual stimuli."[7] Too many intensive care and coronary care units were constructed for the convenience of doctors and nurses, disregarding the detrimental effects on patients.

EFFECTS OF TOUCH

In a study done by McCorkle, it was found that the nurse can establish a rapport with seriously ill patients within a short period of time through touch, which indicates to patients that the nurse cares.[8] Rubin found that in instances of intense personal stress, in which the patient felt isolated and vulnerable, touch comforted and quieted him more quickly than any other mode of communication.[9] Dr. Kubler-Ross, in her work with dying patients, found a most meaningful communication to be gentle pressure of the hand in moments of silence.[10]

Barnett found that registered nurses touch patients almost twice as often as other personnel, and that the areas touched most often were the patient's hand, forehead, and shoulder. Interesting enough, she found that patients in fair and good conditions were touched 70 per cent more frequently than acutely ill patients!!![11]

[7] Ibid, p. 72.
[8] Ruth McCorkle. "Effects of Touch on Seriously Ill Patients," *Nursing Research,* 23 (March–April 1974), 125–132.
[9] Reva Rubin. "The Maternal Touch," *Nursing Outlook,* 11 (Nov. 1963), 828–831.
[10] Elizabeth Kubler-Ross. *On Death and Dying,* New York: Macmillan Publishing Co., Inc., 1969, p. 100.
[11] Kathryn E. Barnett. *The Development of a Theoretical Construct of the Concepts of Touch as They Relate to Nursing,* unpublished doctoral dissertation, North Texas State University, Denton, Texas, 1970, p. 87.

Johnson found that touching patients may have varied meanings to both patient and nurse, depending on culture, background, and maturity.[12]

SUMMARY

To sum up, it has been established that

1. *Both* physiological-physical and emotional support are desirable and necessary to patients' welfare.
2. Emotional support can be given at the same time as physical care is given, through touch, tone of voice, eye contact, body movement, and so on.
3. Emotional support only, without due consideration of physiological needs, may spell disaster to acutely ill patients.
4. Patient-teaching and touch are excellent examples of ways to provide emotional support.

Once nurses grasp the concept of these paragraphs, they will no longer dichotomize their care into *either* physical or psychological-emotional care. Their care should be inclusive of both.

Implications of Stress on the Nurse

Besides her role in nursing the sick, the nurse, in too many instances, is expected to participate in, and to coordinate the activities of other hospital departments, i.e., x-ray, laboratory, dietary, pharmacy, and so on. While the doctors expect their orders to be expedited by the nurse; and the pharmacists' medications to be distributed by the nurse; and the dietician's food to be served by nursing personnel; and the radiology department's x-rays of patients who are conveyed by nursing personnel; and the laboratory's examination of blood, stool, sputa, urine, and so on collected by the nurse—there is left little time for the nurses to nurse the patient! Yet, and ironically, this is the nurse's main commitment! Each department is engaged in its own activity, yet the nurse is engaged in *all!* She is called a "good" nurse when she carries out all of these activities and doesn't complain. Consequently, the time she spends with patients in giving nursing care decreases. Therefore,

---

[12] Betty Sue Johnson. "The Meaning of Touch in Nursing," *Nursing Outlook* (Feb. 1965), 59–60.

more and more of her nursing activities are assigned to ancillary nursing personnel who are unable to use scientific judgment in their care of patients.

In too many instances the nurse is expected to understand everyone else, yet she receives little to no understanding from them. This all leads to frustration and hostility in the nurse, which ultimately leave their mark on her. She soon discovers that she is not doing the job she was prepared to do. To use a time-worn phrase, "The nurse is *not* all things to all people, yet, in actuality, she is *still* expected to be!

Burnout in the Nurse

To take another view, patients in specialized areas, such as the intensive care and coronary care units, require a concerted concern and attention from nurses. All of her attention is directed toward these patients, who, by the extent of their illnesses, are understandably unable to reciprocate any concern for her. The direction of attention is one way. (Perhaps this is a reason why the nurse touches the less acute patient more often than the very ill patient, i.e., she receives some positive feedback from the former.) Who, then, does the nurse draw on in these areas for her *own* fulfillment? Unless there is a special understanding and esprit de corps with her peers, head nurse, supervisor, and/or director of nursing, the nurse could easily become exhausted, both emotionally and physically. She could become "burned out" in this high stress, high human-contact profession.

According to Maslach, "The waste of training and talent in many professions because of burnout is staggering." It's destructive to the patients, to the nurses, and to society. The toll is incalculable because "there's no way to measure its attendant ills such as alcoholism, divorce, mental illness, low productivity, and high absenteeism."[13]

WHAT IS "BURNOUT"?

"When you burnout, your emotional center goes. There's nothing that you really care about. You don't have any optimistic feelings;

---

[13] Michael Putney. "Burnout: A High Price for Caring." *The National Observer* (July 11, 1977), pp. 1, 4.

only negative ones. You don't like the people you work with. You treat them in institutional, routinized, dehumanizing ways."[14]

Burnout can happen to anyone, but it happens most to those for whom caring is part of their business and being. It is difficult for a burned out person to care anymore. Those who might be subjected to the calloused treatment of a burned out person are left angered, embarrassed, demoralized, or humiliated.

HOW CAN BURNOUT BE AVOIDED?

To avoid the tolls of burnout, nurses should be encouraged to leave their work at work, to separate their personal and professional lives. It is also suggested that nurses be transferred out of such high pressured areas at periodic intervals, in order to let them "recharge." The nurse needs to express her *need* for help, and to share her problems with her peers, without being considered a "complainer." Too, the nurse who has an *adequate scientific preparation* for the tasks at hand, as well as a sense of humor, will develop her own sense of worth and will tend to forestall burnout.

Those who suffer most from burnout often had the noblest intentions. Their feelings of guilt and inadequacy are also the greatest. Many nurses who are burned out see themselves as the *cause* of the problems.

In a word, nurses, *too,* are human beings who have needs. A one-way caring system depletes her emotionally, increases and exhausts her stress responses, and sets the stage for unhappiness and stress diseases. How, then, can she *possibly* care for her patients effectively with empathy and compassion?

POSSIBLE SOLUTIONS FOR BURNOUT

In the presence of strong social support systems, social stressors will have only minor effects on health. In some hospitals, steps are being taken to avoid burnout of its nurses. Nursing responsibilities are being given back to nurses, while other hospital departments are assuming their *own* responsibilities. Directors of nursing, supervisors, and head nurses are increasingly supporting their nurses' rights to *nurse.* Nurses are being transferred out of high stress areas, periodically. In many schools of nursing, students are being educated more realisti-

[14] Ibid, pp. 1, 14.

cally for the positions they will be assuming. These are all good starts, however, much *more* needs to be done to protect our nurses.

REFERENCE

Shubin, Seymour. "Burnout: The Professional Hazard You Face in Nursing," *Nursing '78* (July 1978), 22–27.

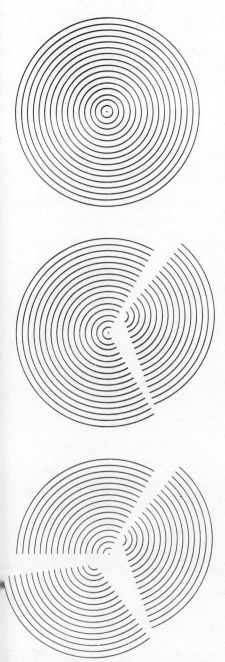

PART III

Patterns of Shock

The direction is forever onward, but the artist still goes back for materials and begins again with the first elements on the most advanced stage; otherwise all goes to ruin.
—*Emerson, "Nature"*

CHAPTER 8

Shock and Major Metabolic Effects

Shock is an abnormal physiological state which is characterized by a disproportion between the circulating blood volume and the size of the diameter of the vascular bed, resulting in circulatory failure and tissue hypoxia. It has been said that hypoxia not only stops the machinery, it wrecks it!

The Three Mechanisms of Shock

The three mechanisms responsible for maintaining circulatory homeostasis are (1) a sufficient blood volume, (2) a healthy heart to pump the blood, and (3) a circulatory vascular system of the right diameter through which the blood can flow under pressure to the capillaries, and return to the right side of the heart. Shock will be induced following the body's inability to compensate for the failure of any one or more of these three mechanisms.

Fortunately, man is equipped with a reserve of internal compensatory (adaptive) mechanisms which provide some degree of protection in delaying the manifestations of shock, i.e., certain mechanisms compensate for a decreasing blood volume, or a failing heart, or excessive dilatation of the peripheral vascular bed. SOME OF THE SIGNS AND SYMPTOMS EXHIBITED BY THE PATIENT ARE THE RESULT OF THESE COMPENSATORY MECHANISMS IN ACTION. These compensatory mechanisms can sustain the patient temporarily. Unless the cause of the circulatory failure is determined and checked, the patient, in all probability, will die.

> PRINCIPLE 30.   Adequate circulation of blood to all body parts is dependent upon a proportionate equilibrium between the blood volume, the strength of cardiac contractions, and the size of the lumina of the vascular bed.

Stages of the general adaptation syndrome

First stage: alarm reaction	Second stage: Stage of resistance	Third stage: stage of exhaustion
Decreasing blood volume, or heart failure, or vasodilatation	The body's efforts to adapt; neuro-endocrine compensatory mechanisms at work	Failure to adapt; compensatory mechanisms fail. Shock results, and, if untreated, death follows.

Shock and the General Adaptation Syndrome

It is through the study of a fascinating subject such as shock that one develops a profound appreciation of the economic and judicious wisdom of the human body, i.e., its wisdom in prolonging life through its economic provision of blood to more vital areas of the body at the expense of less vital parts. One of the nurse's roles is to support the compensatory mechanisms, but unless she understands what they are, she could unwittingly counter their beneficial effects. This, I might add, is done far too often, for instance in the application of heat to the patient in shock. While she must realize the value of the compensatory mechanisms, the nurse must also be aware that the length of time their actions can be sustained is uncertain, and varies from person to person. The nurse who understands these compensatory mechanisms could prolong the stage of resistance, until the deficiency has been replaced and thus prevent the occurrence of shock and possible death.

Another role of the nurse is to expedite therapeutic orders that will assist the patient to cope.

Major Metabolic Effects of Shock on the Body

Discussion of the altered physiology of each type of shock, separately, is not feasible, since there would be needless repetition. Major significant differences, however, will be included in the chapters that follow.

BIOCHEMICAL FEATURES

Regardless of the cause of shock, the following features occur:

↓ Oxygen
↓ Temperature
Hyperglycemia in the initial period
↓ Blood glucose in the late stage
Lactic and pyruvic acidemia
Acidosis (severe shock)
Azotemia
↓ Urine output
↓ Serum sodium and chloride
↑ Serum potassium
↓ Excretion of sodium chloride and water
↓ Vitamin C in the blood
↑ ACTH and adrenal cortical hormones
↑ Adrenal medullary hormones: epinephrine and norepinephrine
↑ ADH (antidiuretic hormone)
Impaired liver function

The prognosis of shock is correlated with the following:

1. The state of consciousness
2. Urinary output
3. Ventilation
4. Liver disease
5. Acid-base balance
6. Age

121

Coma, anuria, and respiratory difficulties are lethal signs, and are associated with a poor prognosis.

A decreased blood pressure is not the principal abnormality in shock, but rather, it is the poor perfusion of the cells with adequate supplies. Hence, there is a gross discrepancy between supply and demand. Blood flow, rather than blood pressure, is the important determinant of survival. An increased blood pressure does not necessarily mean that the tissues are being adequate perfused with blood.

The metabolic abnormalities resulting from shock are secondary changes as a result of decreased blood flow, i.e., decreased delivery of oxygen, nutrients, water, electrolytes, and hormones to the cells, tissues, organs, and systems, and a decreased removal of wastes.

There can be considerable alteration in blood volume, heart pump, and vascular bed while an adequate flow of blood to the tissues continues, as long as compensatory mechanisms are maintained.

THE CELLS

Decreased supply of the five substances to the cells is followed by an initial depression and alteration of cell-function, and eventual cell death which is followed by depressed function of tissues, organs, and systems. The weakened cell membranes predispose to the entrance of sodium and water into the cell, and the exit of potassium from the cell. Because of this abnormal exit of potassium from the cells into the interstitial compartment, the potassium content rises in the interstitial compartment. This is *not* reflected in high potassium levels in the plasma of the vascular compartment, initially. Subsequently, the blood serum potassium levels become high, as the potassium transudes into the vascular compartment.

CENTRAL NERVOUS SYSTEM

An increasing carbon dioxide level in the blood dilates the blood vessels of the brain, thus providing for a sufficient blood supply during the early stages of shock. Progression of shock implies decreased oxygen in the blood, hence the development of cerebral hypoxia. The patient's sensorium is the best indicator of the adequacy of cerebral blood flow. The earliest signs of cerebral hypoxia are restlessness and mental haziness. As the blood pressure continues to decrease, apathy, stupor, semi-consciousness, and coma occur. In the late stages of shock, the subconscious mental functions, including vasomotor and respiratory control, fail.

BLOOD FLOW

The flow of blood is markedly decreased during shock, and is accentuated by stagnant anoxia and capillary stasis. The red blood cells tend to form clumps, often called "sludging." White blood cells adhere to the walls of the venules, thereby further obstructing the flow of the red blood cells. Small clots may form in the small blood vessels.

Systemic blood flow

The most profound metabolic effects of shock occur in the energy pathways of the cells. Hypoperfusion of the cells occurs first in the nonvital tissues, such as the gastrointestinal tract, muscles, connective tissue, and skin. This is compensatory, as the blood is shunted from these less vital parts to the more vital ones. Later, if the shock condition is not checked, hypoperfusion occurs in the vital areas of the brain, heart, lungs, liver, and kidneys. In the late stages of shock, there is decreased flow to the vasomotor center in the brain, which depresses it, rendering it totally inactive. This is followed by marked vascular failure (vasodilatation). Arteriolar dilatation leads to a decreased flow of blood to the heart and brain. Venous dilatation causes increased pooling of blood in the veins, thereby decreasing the return of blood to the right atrium and leading to a subsequent decreased cardiac output. Hypoxia causes increased capillary permeability, therefore, vascular fluid enters and sequesters in the interstitial compartment, further decreasing the circulating blood volume and cardiac output.

CORONARY CIRCULATION AND THE MYOCARDIUM

Normally, coronary circulation is about 5 per cent of the cardiac output. Seventy to 90 per cent of coronary blood-flow occurs during diastole. Consequently, the diastolic blood pressure is important in regulating coronary blood flow. In hemorrhagic shock, if the loss of blood is rapid, coronary insufficiency and myocardial failure will occur early.

Initially, myocardial hypoxia leads to dilatation of the coronary vessels. Epinephrine also dilates the coronary arteries and, indirectly,

123

it increases aortic pressure, thereby increasing coronary flow to the myocardium. In shock there is an impairment of coronary perfusion, due to severe hypotension; hence, myocardial depression and decreased cardiac output follow.

HEART RATE

Initially, there is an increase in heart rate and contractility due to increased sympathetic nervous system stimulation and increased epinephrine. Increased epinephrine and cortisol levels in the blood stream have inotropic and chronotropic effects on the heart, which increases myocardial contractility which, in turn, increases cardiac output. Cortisol secretion is not diminished until the mean blood pressure falls below 35 mm Hg. Adrenocortical failure does not result from circulatory shock. When the venous return of blood to the right atrium decreases, the cardiac output will diminish accordingly.

KIDNEYS, HORMONES, AND BLOOD VESSELS

The kidneys help to maintain the internal stability of the body by excreting a major part of the nitrogenous wastes of protein metabolism, and regulating the volume and tonicity of body fluids. The acid-base balance is preserved by the renal excretion of hydrogen ions, bicarbonate ions, and fixed acids.

Normally, the kidneys produce 12–15 drops of urine per minute (roughly 1 ml.). At least 400 ml. per day of water-excretion is necessary to rid the body of wastes. The major determinants of urine production are the GFR (primarily), and the ability of the tubular cells to reabsorb sodium and glucose. The amounts of antidiuretic hormone and aldosterone also affect the kidneys' ability to retain fluid in the body. With increased ADH and aldosterone there is decreased urine formation.

Renal blood flow is decreased, due to the severe renal arteriolar vasoconstriction caused by the effects of norepinephrine. Urine output decreases to a minimum in an attempt to maintain extracellular fluid volume. Decreased blood to the kidney tissue leads to tubular necrosis. With a loss of nephrons, the patient could die of uremia.

Acute renal insufficiency usually follows shock. Oliguria (less than 350–400 ml. urine per 24 hours) is followed by anuria (less than 20 ml. urine per 24 hours). An increasing blood-urea-nitrogen (BUN) in the presence of adequate hydration and arterial blood pressure indicates acute renal parenchymal damage. Decreased urine output is an indication that the visceral organs are *not* being adequately perfused with blood. In the early stage of shock, peripheral vascular resistance shunts the blood away from the periphery to the visceral organs (including the kidneys) which need it most. If the shock state is not improved, the blood supply to the kidneys will be curtailed.

Decreased flow of blood to the renal parenchyma stimulates the release of renin from the kidneys. Renin leads to the elevation of angiotensin in the blood, which is a potent vasoconstrictor, as well as the most powerful stimulant of aldosterone secretion from the adrenal cortex. Aldosterone conserves sodium, which in turn, conserves water. Increased sodium in the blood, as well as a decreased blood volume, stimulates the release of ADH from the posterior pituitary gland. ADH conserves water, further increasing the blood volume and maintaining the extracellular fluid volume. Aldosterone potentiates the pressor effects of norepinephrine on arterioles, causing increased peripheral resistance and increased cardiac output. The sodium retained tends to enter the arterial walls, and, with it goes water. Together, they decrease the size of the lumina, thereby increasing the arteriolar resistance and blood pressure.

Norepinephrine is a potent alpha adrenergic catecholamine which constricts arterioles and veins. Increased arteriolar resistance (constriction) decreases capillary pressure; hence there is less flow across the capillary membrane. At the venous end of the capillary, the colloid osmotic pressure (C.O.P.) is enhanced, thus a mobilization of fluid from the interstitial compartment into the vascular compartment occurs, and increases the circulating blood volume. If the shock is due to hemorrhage, the colloid osmotic pressure will proportionately decrease with an increasing blood-loss; hence, there will be less mobilization of fluid into the vascular compartment. Initially, however, blood loss is compensated by this mobilization.

Venous constriction, initially, increases the flow of blood to the right atrium, resulting in an increased cardiac output. If, however, venous constriction persists (1) the flow of blood into the right atrium will decrease, and (2) the capillary pressure at the venous end will increase. This will prevent fluid from leaving the interstitial compartment and entering the vascular compartment.

When the sympathetic nervous system and the alpha vasoconstrictors can no longer constrict the blood vessels, a profound vasodilatation occurs. This represents compensatory failure. At this time, the arterioles become markedly dilated, thereby increasing the capillary pressure. As a consequence, fluid pours into the interstitial compartment and it decreases in the vascular compartment. Due to the decreased circulation of blood through the vaso vasorum, the capillaries become weak; hence, the permeability of their membrane is increased. If shock is due to hemorrhage, the loss of whole blood decreases the plasma volume, therefore, the C.O.P. is markedly decreased, the mobilization of fluid from the interstitial compartment ceases. The loss of red blood cells decreases the oxygen-carrying capacity, and weakness of all tissues, and so on ensues, along with increasing anaerobic metabolism and metabolic acidosis. In short, the machinery is wrecked!

BLOOD PRESSURE

In Part One we said that blood pressure is made up of five factors: 1) blood volume, 2) cardiac output, 3) elasticity of the blood vessels, 4) the size of the diameter of the blood vessels, and 5) the viscosity of the blood. In full-blown shock, there is a decreased circulating blood volume, decreased cardiac output, an increased size of the diameter of blood vessels (vasodilatation), and an increased viscosity of the blood.

As peripheral arteriolar resistance decreases (dilatation), the diastolic blood pressure decreases (among other things, the diastolic blood pressure is a measure of peripheral resistance). A decrease in peripheral resistance, which is not compensated by increases in heart rate or stroke volume, results in a lowering of the diastolic blood pressure and an increase (widening) of the pulse pressure.

In uncompensated shock, cardiac output decreases due to decreased return of venous blood to the right atrium, which, in turn, is due to the massive peripheral arteriolar vasodilatation which increases the capillary pressure and floods the interstitial compartment, further lowering the amount of circulating blood. Uncompensated shock is also followed by continuing weakness of the myocardium due to the decreased blood volume and decreased diastolic pressure which directly decrease the flow of blood through the coronary arteries to the myocardium. Treatment must be aimed at (1) restoring the blood volume, (2) strengthening the heart, or (3) restoring the normal luminal size of the blood vessels. Depending on the *cause* of the shock, therapy should revolve around the restoration of any one or more of these three mechanisms.

THE THYROID GLAND

In the initial stages of shock, the thyroid gland secretes increased thyroxine, which increases the heart rate (tachycardia), increases the velocity of blood flow, increases sympathetic nervous activity, sensitizes the tissues to epinephrine, increases the systolic blood pressure, and widens the pulse pressure. On the negative side, thyroxine increases the demands of the tissues for oxygen through its hypermetabolic action.

THE LIVER

Epinephrine causes the liver to release glucose (glucogenolysis) to provide energy nutrients to the nervous system. Normally, the liver is the major site for the conversion of lactate to pyruvate. In shock, there is an accumulation of lactate, which implies a severe impairment of blood flow to the liver and a decreased glycogen content.

TISSUES, ORGANS, AND BODY SYSTEMS

Since shock represents a severe deficiency of oxygen, glucose, water, electrolytes, and hormones to all body cells, the muscle, nerve, connective, and epithelial cells and tissues become markedly weakened if the shock state is not reversed. Then too, the organs and body systems go into a relative state of failure. ALL SIGNS AND SYMPTOMS ARE A REFLECTION OF THE DEFICIENCIES TO CELLS, TISSUES, ORGANS, AND SYSTEMS.

OTHER METABOLIC EFFECTS

Other metabolic effects of shock are the following:

1. Increase in blood concentration of free fatty acids (FFA), due to the gluconeogenesis effects of cortisol.
2. Increased caloric expenditure from 15 to 20 per cent.
3. Acceleration of the synthesis of C-AMP.
4. Decreased body temperature due to decreased blood flow and decreased cardiac output which lead to a decrease of the five substances to the cells, which, in turn, decreases metabolism. Anything that increases the metabolic needs of the cells could hasten the demise of the patient. THE APPLICATION OF EX-

127

TERNAL HEAT SHOULD BE AVOIDED, AS HEAT STIMULATES THE
METABOLIC PROCESS.

5. (Early shock) hyperglycemia from the effects of epinephrine
   and cortisol, leading to glucogenolysis and gluconeogenesis,
   respectively. This protects the brain and heart. However, because there is decreased insulin produced at this time, there
   is decreased oxidation of glucose by the peripheral tissues. It
   is known that catecholamines suppress insulin secretion in any
   form of shock. Perhaps this ensures an adequate amount of
   glucose to the brain, as insulin is not required for the metabolism of glucose by the brian. According to Fleck, however,
   insulin secretion increases later during the same day as the
   occurrence of shock, and may persist for as long as a week.[1]
6. Glucose blood levels rise and insulin decreases with E. Coli
   infections.
7. Burns are followed by decreased insulin production.
8. Glucagon levels increase after injury and burns.
9. After injury, histamine and kinins increase. These increase the
   permeability of cell membranes.

DANGERS OF APPLYING HEAT TO PATIENTS IN SHOCK

EXTERNAL HEAT IS NOT JUSTIFIABLE IN THE TREATMENT OF PA-
TIENTS IN SHOCK. The application of blankets, or any other form of
heat would be detrimental to these patients, with the possible exception
of the severely burned patient. (See section on burn shock.)

In shock, there are decreased supplies of the five substances to
all body cells. The catecholamines have constricted peripheral blood
vessels in order to shunt the blood to the more vital organs. THE APPLI-
CATION OF HEAT WOULD DILATE THE PERIPHERAL ARTERIOLES AND
BRING THE BLOOD FROM THE VISCERAL ORGANS TO THE SKIN. Dilated
arterioles increase the capillary hydrostatic pressure; hence, there is
a further decrease of circulating blood volume, as large quantities of
fluid pour into the interstitial compartment. One degree increase Centigrade in body temperature increases the metabolism by 7 per cent,
thereby creating a greater need for the five substances to the cells.
Heat leads to sweating, which can mean the loss of fluids, potassium,

[1] A. Fleck, "The Early Metabolic Responses" in *Clinical and Experimental Aspects:*
Monographs in Anaesthesiology, Vol. 4, Excerpta Medica, I. Ledingham (ed.), A. R.
Hunter (ed. in chief), New York: American Elsevier Pub. Co., 1976, pp. 57–77.

sodium, and chloride. Only if the patient shivers should external heat be applied, and, in that case, the patient should be covered just enough to stop the shivering. Shivering is caused by rhythmic muscle contractions, therefore, the metabolic effects resemble those of light exercise. Thus, shivering raises the temperature of the skin and leads to cutaneous vasodilatation.

For each degree Centigrade elevation of body temperature, cardiac output and peripheral blood flow increase 25 per cent. Obviously, overheating the patient in cardiogenic shock could hasten his demise.

Baxter, Shires et al., have shown that local renal hypothermia by peritoneal cooling may be a useful adjunct in the treatment of hemorrhagic shock. However, only if the abdomen is opened in the trauma patient with hemorrhagic shock would this be feasible.[2]

INTELLIGENT SENSE VERSUS COMMON SENSE

Intelligent sense, rather than common sense, should be used when the patient in shock tells you that he feels cold. The nurse feels his skin and finds that it *is* cold to her touch. If she uses common sense, she will apply external heat; this is *WRONG!* He feels cold because his compensatory mechanisms have constricted his peripheral blood vessels and shunted the blood to the inner visceral organs. Covering him will only dilate his peripheral vessels and drain the visceral organs by bringing the blood to the skin.

Burton says it quite succinctly: "One change in the older teaching (found particularly in textbooks of nursing) must be made; that is, regarding the dangers of heating the patient in hemorrhagic shock. The dangers of heat are much greater than allowing the patient to be cold, even to the point of hypothermia."[3]

All that needs to be said to the patient is, "I know you feel cool, but I would rather not apply any heat at this time." I might add that heating the patient in shock is *still* a common error among nurses *and* doctors. Despite the fact that it has been proved that overheating the shock patient is dangerous, and that cooling is beneficial, some older practitioners (as well as newer ones), insist that keeping the patient warm is necessary. Our practice must keep abreast with scientific

[2] G. Tom Shires (ed.), *Care of the Trauma Patient,* New York: McGraw-Hill Book Co., 1966, p. 20.
[3] Alan C. Burton, *Physiology and Biophysics of the Circulation,* Chicago: Year Book Medical Publishers, 1965, pp. 201–202.

discoveries. See references on this subject at the end of this chapter. You will notice that one of them is 30 years old!

The Lungs

PULMONARY EDEMA

Dangers of overhydration

Normally, pulmonary interstitial fluid is rapidly drained off by the pulmonary lymphatics which are called the "toilet" of the lungs. Only if their ten-fold normal drainage capacity is exceeded will pulmonary interstitial edema occur. Unless adequate CVP or PAWP monitoring is carried out, there is danger of overloading the circulatory system with intravenous fluids leading to pulmonary edema. This is compounded if the myocardial reserve is marginal, or if acute renal failure is present. Some authorities believe that the lungs are susceptible to pulmonary edema after the infusion of large quantities of noncolloid solutions such as Ringer's Lactate, and other crystalloid solutions. Noncolloid fluids dilute the plasma proteins, thus causing a decreased colloid osmotic pressure in the vascular compartment. As a consequence, more fluid is forced from the arteriolar end of the capillary into the interstitial compartment than is being pulled back into the capillary at the venous end. Hence, large amounts of fluid can become sequestered in the pulmonary interstitial compartment and could transude into the alveoli, decreasing the space for the transfer of oxygen and carbon dioxide. A weakened heart, or renal failure would add to this problem, often referred to as the "wet lung syndrome." In addition, increased capillary permeability in the lungs occurs earlier and is usually more severe than in other body tissues.

The administration of intravenous whole blood, or plasma protein solutions in hemorrhagic shock tends to protect the lungs from the "wet lung syndrome," as they increase the colloid osmotic pressure, hence draw fluid from the pulmonary interstitium back into the blood stream. Pulmonary edema also destroys surfactant which serves as a protection to the alveoli. Monitoring of the patient should be inclusive of accurate intake and output, and daily weights. If patients are breathing high humidity gases, they can absorb large quantites of water through their lungs. A daily chest x-ray during the acute phase of shock will aid in the detection of pleural effusion and pulmonary edema.

Other treatment factors of benefit to the patient with respiratory distress syndrome include:

1. Insertion of an endotracheal tube
2. Diuretics to decrease the amount of fluid in the lungs
3. Albumin, intravenously, to increase the colloid osmotic pressure, and therefore withdraw fluid from the pulmonary interstitial compartment
4. Cardiotonic drugs to increase the efficiency of the heart
5. Corticosteroids to augment the strength of cardiac contractions
6. Antibiotics if the sputum culture is positive
7. Oxygen

INCREASED PULMONARY CAPILLARY PERMEABILITY

All tissues are weakened, due to the decreased oxygen, nutrients, and so on. Increased permeability of the pulmonary capillaries will lead to an escape of large protein molecules (colloids) into the interstitial compartment. Subsequently, large amounts of fluid remain in the interstitial compartment. Examples of causes of increased pulmonary capillary permeability are smoke inhalation, thermal injury, increased histamine, bradykinin and serotonin in allergic states, endotoxic shock, pneumonitis, and fat embolism.

MECHANICAL VENTILATION

All patients on ventilators have a tendency to retain sodium and water. Prolonged mechanical ventilation thus can cause fluid-retention and pulmonary edema. A possible reason for this is that mechanical ventilation increases the antidiuretic hormone, due to the stimulation of volume receptors in the left atrium. An area of the left atrium which adjoins the pulmonary veins is believed to be the site of low pressure volume receptors. Positive pressure respiration and hemorrhage tend to reduce the vagal firing of these receptors, thus resulting in increased ADH secretion from the posterior pituitary gland. When continuous positive pressure ventilation is used in shock patients, there is a danger that CVP measurements may be raised considerably. Other possible causes of fluid-retention and pulmonary edema are fluid-overload and/or subclinical heart failure.

ATELECTASIS (AIRLESS LUNG, OR PART OF A LUNG)

Atelectasis frequently occurs in the shock patient. A prevalent cause is the retention of mucous secretions in the respiratory tract, causing plugging of small bronchioles. If the patient has had surgery, he will most likely have an overproduction and an underelimination of mucous secretions in his tracheal-bronchial tree. Endotracheal anesthesia, by pressing against the inner tracheal wall, often stimulates the mucous glands of the trachea. An underhydrated state and atropine tend to increase the viscosity of these secretions. Morphine dulls the cough reflex, and the patient has no desire to cough. This results in the retention of copious amounts of thick secretions in the tracheal-bronchial tree. If the bronchioles are obstructed, oxygen cannot get into the alveoli to diffuse into the blood stream and carbon dioxide cannot diffuse from the blood stream into the alveoli; hence, an arteriovenous shunt occurs. This results in an admixture of venous and arterial blood, i.e., the carbon dioxide mixes with the arterial blood and a state of hypercapnea exists. An increased amount of carbon dioxide in the arterial blood implies a decreased amount of oxygen. Therefore, the supply of oxygen to all cells of the body will be decreased further. Warm humidification helps to prevent the secretions from becoming encrusted. However, 100 per cent oxygen concentrations should be avoided, as this depresses ciliary motion in the trachea. The patient should be protected from aspirating vomitus. Nasal-tracheal suctioning should be done. When feasible, the patient should be encouraged to clear his throat, take deep sighing breaths every half hour, and cough. Coughing helps to loosen secretions and increase ciliary motion. (Laughing is also useful in the prevention of atelectasis, however, in such a situation there is little reason for the patient to laugh.)

If the patient is receiving a beta adrenergic stimulating drug, such as isoproterenol, he should be observed for excessive secretions which could further block the airway. Other measures to prevent or treat atelectasis are the relief of pain to prevent splinting of the chest, and frequent changes of position. Unless contraindicated, the patient should be turned from side to side every half hour. Caution must be taken not to cause the Valsalva maneuver.

If at all possible, patient-teaching should be done *before* the patient has an operation. Coughing, deep breathing, sighing, and clearing of the throat should all be demonstrated. Unless contraindicated (due to the patient's condition), the patient should be requested to return the demonstrations. Simple explanations that these will aid his breathing, prevent pneumonia, and a collapsed lung are absolutely necessary. The preoperative patient who understands will be more cooperative postoperatively, and, in all probability, will avoid the hazards of atelectasis and pneumonia. Postural drainage, vibratory clapping, high humidity inspirations, broncho-dilators, and mucolytics are other means of preventing and/or treating atelectasis.

Disturbances of Acid-Base Balance

Decreased perfusion of the tissues leads to anaerobic metabolism and metabolic acidosis. Decreased oxygen to the cells leads to cell and cell-membrane damage; hence, lactic acid and serum enzymes accumulate as a result of anaerobic metabolism. At first, the respiratory rate increases (hyperventilation) in a compensatory effort (if the lungs are not obstructed) to decrease the carbon dioxide tension and to prevent the pH of the blood from going to dangerously low levels. (Because of this, *alkalosis* can occur initially in shock.) As metabolic acidosis increases, respiratory compensation will fail and the pH of the blood will decrease. Treatment includes oxygen and buffers. Sodium bicarbonate, an alkalizing solution, is usually given to counter the effects of acidosis. Measurements of the blood pH, pCo_2, and pO_2 are indicated. In late shock there will be increased serum calcium, since calcium ionizes in an acid medium. In traumatized muscle areas and necrotic tissue, serum calcium may fall, due to the trapping of calcium in the injured area. Sodium, normally found in the extracellular fluid and plasma, enters the cells and potassium leaves the cells. Therefore, hyponatremia and hyperpotassemia occur.

THE BOHR EFFECT OF ACIDOSIS

1. The vasomotor tone: There is a biphasic effect; vasoconstriction is followed by vasodilation. Epinephrine and norepinephrine are ineffective in an acidotic medium, hence their ability to constrict peripheral blood vessels diminishes, and vasoconstriction is replaced by vasodilatation.

2. Sodium and water enter the cells and the cells swell. As sodium enters, potassium leaves the cells. This produces a relative hyperpo-

tassemia, especially if oliguria is present. If additional potassium is given at this time, diastolic cardiac arrest may occur.

3. Increased capillary permeability, especially in the intestine. As a consequence, bacteria and endotoxins are absorbed into the blood stream and accentuate the shock condition.

4. The affinity of hemoglobin for oxygen is decreased, and oxygen transport may be impaired; therefore, decreased oxygen leads to increased blood-viscosity and increased clot formation.

5. The effect on the respiratory center is biphasic, with stimulation followed by depression of respirations.

6. If a high blood lactate, a low pH of the blood, and low bicarbonate levels appear early in shock a poor outcome is indicated. Acidosis decreases the irritability and contractile force of the myocardium, leading to a decreased cardiac output. Probably the most important problem presented by severe acidosis is the propensity to cardiac arrest, or ventricular fibrillation.

A wide variety of acid-base abnormalities can occur in critically ill and injured patients. For example:

1. Respiratory alkalosis can occur early in shock, due to hyperventilation of the patient. The blood pH increases. Extreme degrees of hyperventilation may be due to (a) pain, (b) anxiety, hysteria, sepsis, and trauma. In alkalosis, there is a decrease of ionized calcium in the blood, which leads to increased neuromuscular irritability and/or tetany. Treatment is based on frequent blood gases and acid-base measurements. Other causes can be the administration of alkaline substances, excessive losses of gastric secretions, and hypokalemia.

2. Metabolic acidosis usually follows the alkalotic state. This is due to hypoxia of the cells and increased $pCO2$ levels, which are due, directly, to decreased circulation of blood. There is increased lactic acidemia, increased $CO2$, and eventual depression of the respiratory center.

3. Combined respiratory and metabolic acidosis due to decreased oxygen. The blood pH decreases. The patient is restless, has decreased breath sounds, increasing rales, and cyanosis. Hypercapnea develops, due to the shunting of blood in pulmonary capillaries. Unventilated areas of the lungs cause alveolar collapse (atelectasis). Respiratory assistance and blood gases are very useful at this time.

134

THE FOUR UNCOMPENSATED ACID-BASE DISTURBANCES

The four uncompensated acid-base disturbances are:

1. Respiratory alkalosis. This results from hyperventilation and is characterized by decreased pCO_2, slightly decreased HCO_3, and increased pH of the blood.
2. Respiratory acidosis. This is caused by inadequate pulmonary ventilation and is characterized by increased pCO_2, slightly increased HCO_3, and decreased pH of the blood.
3. Metabolic alkalosis. This can result from the loss of hydrochloric acid by vomiting, or from the infusion of excessive amounts of bicarbonate solution. It is also commonly observed after major surgery and is usually due to a loss of hydrochloric acid through gastric suctioning, increased bicarbonate regeneration by the kidneys, and the administration of large amounts of blood. Metabolic alkalosis is characterized by increased HCO_3, normal pCO_2, and increased pH of the blood.
4. Metabolic acidosis. In the shock patient, metabolic acidosis is due to increased blood lactic acid resulting from poor tissue perfusion. Massive blood transfusions are a common cause of metabolic acidosis; citrate intoxication, hypocalcemia and potassium toxicity can result. Metabolic acidosis is characterized by decreased HCO_3, normal pCO_2, decreased pH of the blood, and reduced CO_2 tension.

REFERENCES

Apperly, Frank L. *Patterns of Disease.* Philadelphia: J. B. Lippincott Co., 1951.

Baker, Patrick J. "Postoperative Atelectasis." *Nursing Digest* (Spring 1977). Vol. V, No. 1, pp. 42–44.

Barcenas, C., T. Fuller, and J. Knockel. "Metabolic Alkalosis After Blood Transfusion." *Journal of the American Medical Association,* 236 (Aug. 23, 1976), 953–954.

Baue, A. E. "Metabolic Abnormalities of Shock." *Surgical Clinics of North America,* 56 (Oct. 1976), 1059–1071.

Chaffee, Ellen E., and Esther M. Greisheimer. *Basic Physiology and Anatomy,* 3rd ed. Philadelphia: J. B. Lippincott Co., 1974.

Clowes, George H. A., T. O'Donnell, G. Blackburn, and T. Maki. "Energy Metabolism and Proteolysis in Traumatized and Septic Man." *Surgical Clinics of North America,* 56 (Oct. 1976), 1169–1184.

Cole, Warren H. "Treatment of Surgical Shock" in *Textbook of Surgery,* 7th ed. New York: Appleton-Century-Crofts Co., 1959.

Cunningham, Joseph H., Robert H. Richardson, and Jan D. Smith. "Interstitial Pulmonary Edema." *Heart and Lung,* 6 (July–Aug. 1977), 617–623.

Guyton, Arthur C. *Medical Physiology,* 5th ed. Philadelphia: W. B. Saunders Co., 1976.

Pierce, E. Converse III. "Is Acid-Base Important?" *Medical Times,* 95 (Dec. 1967).

Sodeman, William A., and William A. Sodeman, Jr. *Pathologic Physiology,* 5th ed. Philadelphia: W. B. Saunders Co., 1974.

Thal, Alan P., E. Brown, A. Hermreck, and H. Bell. *Shock: A Physiologic Basis for Treatment.* Chicago: Year Book Medical Publishers, 1971.

Webb, Watts R. *A Protocol for Managing the Pulmonary Complications of Patients in Shock.* Upjohn Co., 1975.

Weil, Max H., and Herbert Shubin. *Diagnosis and Treatment of Shock.* Baltimore: Williams & Wilkins Co., 1967.

Wilson, Robert F. "Acid-Base Abnormalities in Clinical Shock" in William Schumer and Lloyd Nyhus (Eds.). *Treatment of Shock: Principles and Practice.* Philadelphia: Lea and Febiger, 1974, chap. 3.

CHAPTER 9

Hypovolemic Shock

Hypovolemic shock means shock due to the loss of excessive amounts of body fluid. This is inclusive of the following:

A. External Fluid Losses
   1. Hemorrhage (external or internal)
   2. Vomiting
   3. Diarrhea
   4. Renal
      a. Diabetes mellitus
      b. Diabetes insipidus
      c. Excessive use of diuretics
   5. Skin
      a. Burns
      b. Copious perspiration without replacement of fluids
B. Internal Sequestration of Fluid
   1. Fractures
   2. Ascites
   3. Intestinal obstruction
   4. Hemothorax or hemoperitoneum

The overall implications of hypovolemic shock are

Decreased blood volume
   ↓ (leading to)
Decreased venous return to the right heart
   ↓
Decreased cardiac output
   ↓
Decreased tissue perfusion

This type of shock results when the blood volume becomes markedly decreased, and therefore, inadequate to meet the metabolic needs of the body. Any condition that can cause a marked reduction in the blood volume can cause hypovolemic shock. Important examples of some of these conditions are presented in this chapter:

Hemorrhagic shock: a loss of whole blood
Trauma: a loss of whole blood, or plasma
Burn shock: a loss of plasma, primarily
Diabetic acidosis: a loss of fluid and electrolytes from all three fluid compartments
Bowel obstruction: a loss of fluid and electrolytes

Hemorrhagic Shock

In most instances, loss of 30 to 50 per cent of the blood volume in a young previously healthy person results in circulatory failure and manifestations of profound shock. In hemorrhagic shock, if the loss of blood is gradual, over a period of days, compensatory expansion of the plasma volume will prevent acute circulatory failure. If the loss of blood is less than 100 ml. per day, increased erythrocyte formation will compensate fully, and a normal amount of red blood cells will be maintained if the iron stores are sufficient. When the blood loss is more than 100 ml. per day, there will be a slow decrease of red blood cells with a compensatory increase in the plasma volume. The clinical features of the patient will be those of anemia, rather than hypovolemia or shock.

ARTERIAL VERSUS VENOUS BLEEDING

In comparison to arterial hemorrhage, venous hemorrhage behaves differently. Arterial bleeding is characterized by spurts of rapid bleeding. With venous bleeding, the loss of blood is slow but steady, and, of course, it is distal to the capillary-arteriolar bed. Although a decrease in blood pressure occurs, it is readily maintained by an increased peripheral arteriolar and venous vasoconstriction. Peripheral vasoconstriction of the arterioles and venules maintains the blood pressure near normal, and also permits adequate coronary perfusion. Eventually, however, there is a decrease in venous return to the heart which leads to a decrease in the pulmonary inflow, and hence decreased alveolar oxygenation of the blood. Despite this, sufficient oxygenation takes place, arteriolar pressure is maintained by vasoconstriction, and there is an adequate perfusion of the coronary blood vessels. Therefore, the patient is able to tolerate shock from venous hemorrhage better than from hemorrhage of a large artery.

Major Implications of Hemorrhagic Shock

Hemorrhagic shock implies loss of red blood cells and plasma. Considering that the five substances necessary for cell health and metabolism are carried in the whole blood, the major implication of hemorrhage, then, is a decrease of supplies to the four types of body cells, namely, muscle, nerve, connective, and epithelial. Signs and symptoms derive from this. Since an adequate blood volume is necessary for the removal of cell wastes, there is decreased elimination of these wastes; hence an increased accumulation in the cells and tissues.

Decreased plasma implies decreased fluid, electrolytes, and colloid osmotic pressure (C.O.P.). With a decreased C.O.P. there is a decreased osmotic pulling power of fluids from the interstitial compartment into the vascular compartment; hence, fluid is sequestered in the interstitial compartment, and the compensatory osmosis to increase the blood volume is temporarily lost. Since plasma also contains water and sodium, a severe deficiency of these may occur.

As red blood cells and plasma are lost during hemorrhage, neither the hemoglobin nor the hematocrit are of direct aid as measurements of blood volume. When interstitial fluid is eventually mobilized into the vascular compartment (due to increased arteriolar constriction), the hemoglobin and hematocrit are diluted. A continued fall in hematocrit after 24–36 hours almost certainly signifies progressive bleeding.

BLOOD FLOW VERSUS BLOOD PRESSURE

There is increasing recognition that shock is due to a failure of blood-flow and tissue perfusion, rather than to a failure of blood pressure. Initially in shock, peripheral vasoconstriction maintains the blood flow. With increasing vasoconstriction less blood enters the capillaries, and there is inadequate cellular perfusion of the five substances carried by the blood. This implies a decrease to the capillaries of the skin, brain, kidneys, and heart.

One should not rely solely on blood pressure readings, but rather on the *changes* in both systolic and diastolic readings, and, mainly, on the direct observation of the patient. Too often, nurses rely on the blood pressure without taking the physical and mental aspects of the patient into proper consideration. Whenever possible, the nurse should know, and record for ready reference, the patient's normal blood pressure. Although this is not usually available in the emergency room, it *is* available for other hospital patients who have their blood pressures checked on admission. Although this blood pressure reading may be a little higher than normal (due to stress), it is usually more accurate than a preoperative reading. Many times the preoperative blood pressure is taken after the patient has been medicated for surgery.

FRACTURES AND HYPOVOLEMIA

Open fractures often lead to hemorrhage, which may occur from a major artery cut by a bony fragment. Open fractures of the femur and proximal tibia are especially prone to considerable hemorrhage. Closed fractures can also cause shock as a result of internal bleeding and loss of extracellular fluid from the circulating blood volume. The loss of blood into the tissues as a result of fractures of the pelvis, spine, or femur should not be underestimated. As much as 1000–1500 ml. of whole blood, and the same amount of extracellular fluid may be lost into the tissues of the thigh from a closed comminuted fracture of the femoral shaft, along with the injury of the soft tissue.

Hemorrhage from open fractures of the extremities can usually be controlled by a compression dressing. However, the loss of blood into the tissues from a fractured pelvis or spine cannot be controlled as readily. Blood transfusions of sufficient quantity are indicated promptly. Isotonic saline solutions are also usually indicated.

BONE INJURY AND FAT EMBOLI

One of the most serious complications of traumatic bone injury is fat embolism. The fat embolism syndrome may also develop in the absence of any trauma, such as in association with diabetes, burns, infections, inhalation anesthesia, metabolic disorders, neoplasms, osteomyelitis, blood transfusions, cardiopulmonary bypass, renal infarction, and homotransplantation, steroid-induced fatty liver, and sickle cell illness.

Embolization of fat can occur throughout the pulmonary vascular bed, and is related to the fracture of bones containing the most marrow, such as long bones, ribs, and pelvis. In the pulmonary circulation, the fat blocks the capillaries and causes hemorrhagic interstitial pneumonitis. As a result of this, the following can develop: (1) an impairment of the alveolar-capillary exchange, leading to hypoxia, and (2) pulmonary interstitial edema and hemorrhage.

Major signs and symptoms of fat embolization are as follows:

1. Behavior changes, disorientation. Striking changes in the mental state resulting in restlessness, confusion, and belligerence are often the first indication of the fat embolism syndrome.
2. Increasing pulse rate and temperature.
3. Blood pressure is usually normal.
4. Tachypnea, dyspnea, bubbly rales, and wheezing.
5. Superficial vein fullness due to increased venous pressure may be present.
6. Petechial rash appears two to three days after injury. This rash usually appears on the anterior chest, axillae and clavicular areas, and does not blanch with pressure. The rash is possibly due to embolization of skin vessels.

IMPLICATIONS FOR TREATMENT

Treatment of the patient with fat emboli includes the following:

1. Do not move patient
2. Tracheostomy, assisted ventilation, suctioning PRN, O2
3. Corticosteroids
4. Heparin to lower the plasma proteins and increase the flow of the microcirculation

141

5. Low molecular weight dextran to decrease the aggregation of the erythrocytes and to improve capillary flow
6. Relief of pain and apprehension

IMPLICATIONS OF A DECREASED BLOOD VOLUME ON THE HEART

The left side of the heart can only pump into the circulation the amount of blood it receives from the right side of the heart. Initially, during the loss of blood volume, the sympathetic nervous system and the action of the adrenergic vasoconstrictors provide for an adequate venous return and left ventricular output. Unless the *cause* of the decreased volume is determined and checked, there will be a decreased return of venous blood to the right side of the heart, and therefore a decreased cardiac output. A major implication of this on the myocardium is a decreased amount of blood-flow through the coronary blood vessels to the myocardial muscle. Although decreased oxygen and adrenergic agents dilate the coronary vessels, compensatorily, if the patient is not treated, coronary and myocardial weakness and insufficiency—with a consequent decreased cardiac output—will ensue.

State of consciousness

Unconsciousness is not common in the patient in hemorrhagic shock. Before he becomes unconscious, the patient is usually in very deep shock with a loss of half or more of his normal blood volume. Unconsciousness following blood loss *and* trauma may be due to intracranial injury, rather than to blood loss.

THE HEMORRHAGING PATIENT AND GENERAL ANESTHESIA

The hemorrhaging patient is especially vulnerable to the effects of general anesthetics. Commonly used inhalation anesthetics, with the exception of nitrous oxide, exert a depressant effect on the myocardium, thereby decreasing the cardiac output. Even though the patient may be in compensated shock, he can develop a profound and fatal hypotension when general anesthetics are given, as these agents can also cause a depression of the peripheral homeostatic mechanism, thereby dilating the peripheral blood vessels. In addition, general anesthetics can accentuate acidosis, which the hypovolemic patient may already have.

142

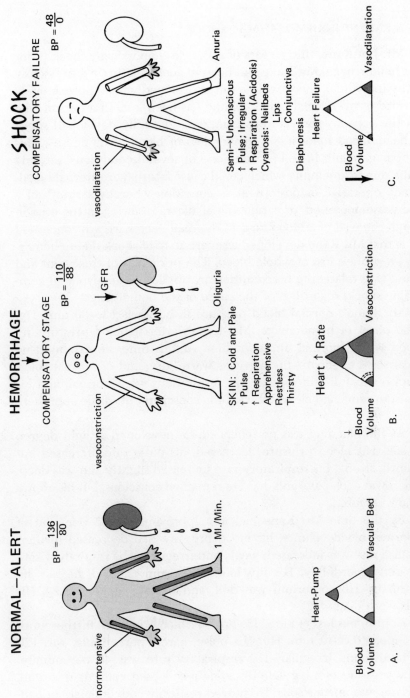

Figure 17. A. Dynamic equilibrium of blood volume, heart pump and vascular bed.
B. Decreased blood volume. Compensation by heart pump and vascular bed.
C. Further decrease in blood volume. Compensatory failure of heart and vascular bed.

143

A PATIENT IN HEMORRHAGIC SHOCK

Mr. Jim Kane, thirty years of age, is in hemorrhagic shock. Prior to his hemorrhage, Mr. Kane had been in good health. (In a previously healthy individual, shock will be fully developed when approximately one third of his normal blood volume has been lost. In a person who lacks the capacity for vigorous compensation, fully developed shock will be induced following a smaller loss of blood.) The cause of his hemorrhage could have been any one of several conditions, i.e., any trauma due to any injury which could cause internal or external bleeding, any operative or postoperative condition whereby a suture of a blood vessel loosened, or carcinoma or ulcers resulting in the erosion through the wall of a blood vessel. The main factor we are concerned with is that Mr. Kane developed a severe state of shock due to hemorrhage, a profuse loss of whole blood. The principles of treatment and nursing care relating to his condition are applicable to anyone in hemorrhagic shock, regardless of the cause of the hemorrhage.

Mr. Kane's normal blood pressure in health is 136/80 mm. Hg. At the onset of hemorrhage, Mr. Kane's arterial blood pressure remained within normal limits for him. At this time, he exhibited no clinical signs of shock—his skin was warm, dry, and of normal color, his pulse was full and regular, his respirations were normal, and his sensorium remained clear. He was fully conscious but a little apprehensive.

As the bleeding was not checked, he developed a slight degree of shock. His blood pressure decreased, his pulse rate increased but was fairly strong, his respiratory rate increased slightly and was deep. His skin was cool, pale, and dry. He remained conscious, but his apprehension persisted.

By the time Mr. Kane had lost approximately 35 per cent of his normal blood volume, his blood pressure had decreased further. His pulse rate was increased, weak, and irregular. His respiratory rate increased accordingly. His lips looked dry and cracked; he said he was thirsty. His sensorium was dull, and he said he felt dizzy. His pupils were dilated.

Continuous loss of blood lowered his blood pressure further, until it dropped to 68/0 mm. Hg. His pulse, barely perceptible, was 120 per minute and irregular. His respiratory rate was 40 per minute. Digital pressure of a leg vein disclosed a collapsed vein. At this time, Mr. Kane was unconscious. He moved restlessly and aimlessly in bed.

His skin was cold, clammy, and of an ashen gray hue. There was frank cyanosis of his lips and fingernail beds. His urinary output by indwelling catheter was nil at this time.

Let us trace the signs and symptoms exhibited by Mr. Kane from the onset and compensated stage of hemorrhage to a later uncompensated stage of shock. Bear in mind that in the following clinical picture, the fundamental feature is a persisting deficiency in the blood supply to the tissues, due to the loss of blood volume and, eventually, to a failure of the compensatory mechanisms of which vasoconstriction plays a dominant role in this situation. For obvious purposes of this text, Mr. Kane's clinical course extends from the onset of hemorrhage to a severe state of shock. The provision of effective treatment, i.e., the replacement of his blood volume and the stoppage of bleeding from its source, could reverse his clinical course at any time—with the possible exception of the period of severe shock, which could terminate in irreversible shock, and, consequently, in death.

Blood loss and relative degree of shock*

Degree of clinical severity of shock	Approximate amount of blood lost (per cent of normal value)	Systolic blood pressure (Mr. Kane's normal blood pressure: 136/80)	Decrease in blood pressure (per cent of normal)
No clinical signs of shock	15	132/82	3
Slight degree of shock	20	110/88	20
Moderately severe shock	35	86/50	35
Severe shock	45	68/0	50

* Adapted from the range of percentages given by H. K. Beecher et al.: "The Internal State of the Severely Wounded Man on Entry to the Most Forward Hospital." *Surgery,* 22 (1947), 672–711.

In the practice of nursing, it is rare not to be exposed at some time to patients in each of the degrees of shock portrayed in the following clinical situation. The nurse's first encounter with the hemorrhaging patient is not always at the time when he is beginning to lose blood; for example, if the bleeding is the result of an accident, by the time the person is brought to the hospital, his degree of shock could be in any of the stages mentioned below.

The following format includes two columns; the first column includes the signs and symptoms, which answer the question *What?* The second column includes physiologic explanations, which answer the question *Why?* Compensatory mechanisms are also included in column two.

Signs and symptoms (what?)	*Physiological explanations* (why?) *and compensatory mechanisms*
Onset of hemorrhage Approximately 15% loss of total blood volume. No clinical signs of shock. BP = 132/82; within a normal range of Mr. Kane's normal BP of 136/80. Blood gases and pH normal. Place patient in a supine position, with legs elevated. 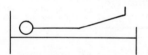 Pulse 80/min., strong and regular. Resp. 22/min. Check patient's airway. Make sure it is patent. Suction PRN.	The normal blood volume is about 7% of the lean body weight. (Blood loss is commonly underestimated, for example, a count and weighing of blood-soaked sponges in the operating room ignores losses of the blood or plasma that has abnormally entered the tissues). Even though the blood volume is decreasing, the BP is often maintained within the normal limits for awhile. This is due to the compensatory mechanisms, i.e., the sympathetic nervous system and the catecholamines, epinephrine and norepinephrine. The most potent stimuli of epinephrine and norepinephrine are hemorrhage, oligemic shock, hypoxia, and certain psychological stimuli such as excitement and fear. The initial constriction of the veins by norepinephrine increases the return of blood to the heart. This is often 2½ fold, as the veins are a reservoir for blood. The slight increase in diastolic pressure indicates the degree of arteriolar constriction, due to norepinephrine. At this time, arteriolar vasoconstriction leads to a decreased capillary hydrostatic pressure, so less fluid crosses the capillary membrane into the interstitial area. Hence, the colloid osmotic pressure is enhanced at the venous end of the capillary, and large amounts of fluid begin to enter the capillary from the interstitial compartment, in an effort to swell the blood volume; hence, compensating for the volume deficit for awhile. Hypoxia stimulates the red bone marrow, therefore, more red blood cells are released into the circulation. With the increased number of red blood

Signs and symptoms (what?)	Physiological explanations (why?) and compensatory mechanisms
	cells, more oxygen-carrying power is made available. When red cell formation occurs at an abnormally rapid rate, immature red cells pass into the blood stream. Since immature red cells contain less hemoglobin, there will be less oxygen-carrying power. Anoxia also stimulates erythropoietin, an erythropoiesis-stimulating factor which is produced or activated in the kidneys. After acute hypoxia or bleeding, an increased concentration of erythropoietin is detected in the plasma.
Conscious.	Consciousness indicates that the brain is receiving a sufficient blood supply.
CVP = 5 cm. H2O pressure (normal).	A CVP line was inserted in the superior vena cava; the normal pressure of which is 6–8 cm. H2O. (The CVP falls approximately 0.7 cm. H2O per 100 ml. of blood loss in a 70 kg. subject. When successive CVP measurements show a progressive decline, continuing blood-loss should be suspected.)
PWP (Pulmonary wedge pressure) normal; 16 cm. H2O.	A normal PWP indicates that the left cardiac performance is satisfactory at this time.
Temperature 98.4.	Slightly below normal, indicating a slightly decreased metabolic rate.
Pulse 86/min. (rising).	Due to the sympathetic nervous system and epinephrine, the heart rate is increasing. (See p. 41 on counting the pulse.)
Slight degree of shock Approximately 20% loss of total blood volume. BP = 110/88, the systolic BP is approximately 20% below his normal. CVP = 3 mm. Hg. Urine output satisfactory.	The systolic BP begins to decline when the total blood volume is decreased by about 15–20% of normal. (It is not unusual for some people to lose as much as 25% of their total blood volume without exhibiting any signs of shock.) The decreased systolic BP indicates that the venous return of blood to the heart is decreasing; therefore, a decreased cardiac output. This could be due to sustained venous constriction, as well as to a decreasing blood volume. The diastolic pressure is greater than before, indicating increasing arteriolar constriction. The degree of, and length of constriction varies from per-

147

Signs and symptoms (what?)	Physiological explanations (why?) and compensatory mechanisms
	son to person. The circulation continues to operate almost normally, even when as much as 25% of the total blood volume has been lost.
Temperature 98.2.	Decreased temperature indicates a slight decline in metabolism.
Pulse rate increasing, 88/min. and fairly strong.	The heart rate is increased due to epinephrine and the sympathetic nervous system, and also through the stimulation of the carotid and aortic reflexes. Due to increased heart rate and the constricted arteries, the crest and ebb of the pulse occur more frequently. An increased heart rate implies increased myocardial work which provides the muscle power for cardiac contraction. Epinephrine and decreased oxygen dilate the coronary blood vessels through which an increased amount of blood flows to the myocardium to meet its needs. Cortisol's inotropic effect on the heart increases its contractile force.
Hyperglycemia.	Due to increased epinephrine which stimulates the liver to release glucose (glucogenolysis). Since epinephrine does not stimulate insulin production, the glucose is not metabolized by the peripheral cells. Presumably (?), the elevated glucose level in the blood serves as a protection of the brain (the most vital part of the body), since brain cells metabolize glucose *without* the presence of insulin.
Respiratory rate increased 24/min.	Decreased blood volume implies decreased red blood cells and hemoglobin which, in turn, implies decreased oxygen-carrying power, resulting in minor cellular hypoxia at this time. Decreased hemoglobin also implies decreased carbon dioxide carrying-power. However, since carbon dioxide diffuses twenty times faster than oxygen in the lungs, the retention of carbon dioxide is not a problem at this time. Compensatorily, the carbon dioxide stimulates the respiratory center in the medulla oblongata of the brain.
Skin pale, cool, and dry. (Pallor in brown skin ap-	Due to the shunting of blood from the periphery to the viscera there is less blood in the

Signs and symptoms (what?)	Physiological explanations (why?) and compensatory mechanisms
pears yellowish-brown, and in the black skin it appears ashen gray.)	skin vessels. Oxygenated arterial blood gives color and warmth to the skin; hence, Mr. Kane's skin is pale and cool. IT IS IMPORTANT THAT THE PATIENT *NOT* BE OVERHEATED (UNLESS HE SHIVERS), AS HEAT WILL (1) DILATE PERIPHERAL BLOOD VESSELS AND BRING THE BLOOD FROM THE VISCERA TO THE SKIN, (2) INCREASE METABOLISM, HENCE INCREASING THE NEED FOR OXYGEN, AND SO ON, TO THE CELLS, (3) IMPOSE A BURDEN ON THE HEART TO INCREASE ITS PUMPING, AND (4) CAUSE SWEATING, THEREFORE, THE LOSS OF FLUID AND ELECTROLYTES.
Do not apply heat. *If patient shivers, cover lightly until the shivering stops.*	
Conscious, apprehensive and restless	While consciousness is maintained, there is a decreased amount of blood going to the brain, as is evidenced by restlessness.
BP = 98/70 M.A.P. = 79 mm. Hg. Oliguric. Urine output 24 ml. during last hour.	With oliguria and anuria, K+ is trapped in the blood stream. Signs of K + excess are twitching, and irregular pulse due to an irritable heart muscle; cramps, nausea, and diarrhea. A decreased urine volume is often the earliest sign of hypovolemia.
Patient says he is thirsty. Lips dry and cracked. Dry mucous membranes.	Thirst indicates cellular dehydration. During the course of shock, large amounts of fluid leave the cells and interstitial compartment and enter the vascular compartment.
Moderately severe shock Approximately 35% loss of total blood volume.	
BP = 86/50 M.A.P. = 63 mm. Hg.	Mr. Kane continues to lose blood, while his sympathetic nervous system, epinephrine, norepinephrine, aldosterone, cortisol, antidiuretic hormone, and angiotensin are still trying to compensate for his decreased blood volume, their concerted efforts are not sufficient at this time. Note that his diastolic pressure is declining, an indication of decreased norepinephrine and decreased vasomotor stimulation to the muscle layer of his peripheral blood vessels. A relative degree of arteriolor and venous dilatation occurs. The systolic pressure is declining, due to the decreased venous return.
Anuric.	Mr. Kane's mean arterial pressure is only 63 mm. Hg. pressure, and is not sufficient for

149

Signs and symptoms (what?)	*Physiological explanations* (why?) and compensatory mechanisms
	the production of urine, as it takes at least 70 mm. Hg. for this to occur. No urine output indicates that the hemorrhage is continuing. We also know that the important visceral organs are not being adequately perfused with blood. At this time there will be increasing signs of visceral organ failure.
CVP = 4 cm. H₂O.	Since CVP measures the competency of the right heart to pump the blood, a CVP reading of 4 cm. H₂O indicates that intravenous fluid can be given fairly rapidly. The fluid of choice is whole blood.

Laboratory data:
  Decreased rbc
  Decreased plasma
    proteins
  Hyperglycemia
  Decreased blood pH
Decreased pO2
  Increased pCO2
  Increased lactic
    acids

Nail beds light bluish;
  skin pale.

Respiratory rate increasing,
  36/min.

Pulse rate 104/min., irregular.

Patient remains conscious.
  Restless and apprehensive.

Loss of whole blood implies the loss of red blood cells and plasma. Therefore, there is decreased oxygen-carrying power of the hemoglobin in the red cells. A relative state of hypoxia occurs. Decreased plasma proteins indicates decreased colloid osmotic pressure; hence, the mobilization of fluids from the interstitial compartment into the vascular compartment decreases markedly. Coupled with increased arteriolar dilatation (which increases capillary hydrostatic pressure) mobilization of fluid ceases. Compensatory failure continues. Decreased blood pH, increased pCO2, decreased PO2, and increased lactic acids indicate metabolic acidosis. An increased respiratory rate is attempting to compensate for this.

Hyperglycemia is due to the release of glucose from the liver (glucogenolysis caused by increased epinephrine and cortisol). Since insulin is not produced at this time, a high blood glucose level occurs.

The sympathetic nervous system and epinephrine increase the heart rate. Too much epinephrine can cause cardiac arrhythmias; hence irregularity of the pulse.

In a supine position with legs elevated 30 degrees, sufficient oxygen is getting to Mr. Kane's brain to sustain consciousness. However, restlessness and apprehension indicate

Signs and symptoms (what?)	*Physiological explanations* (why?) *and compensatory mechanisms*
	that there is a relative decrease in oxygen to the brain. There is a deficiency of blood,
Weakness	therefore, a decreased amount of the five substances to the cells (O_2, H_2O, glucose,
Lab. Increased FFA (free fatty acids).	electrolytes, and hormones) leading to weakness of muscle, nerve, connective, and epithelial cells. Gluconeogenesis—the breakdown of tissues into glucose—is occurring from the action of cortisol, in an effort to increase energy.
Pulse rate 108/min.	Cardiac function is usually not impaired until the later stages of shock. However, in the event of any signs of heart failure, digitalization may be prescribed to aid myocardial function. The quantity of blood ejected by the heart depends on (1) the amount of blood that enters the ventricles during diastole, (2) the force of cardiac contractions, and (3) the heart rate. Insults to the heart by the low blood volume imply (1) decreased amount of blood entering the ventricles because of decreased volume and decreased venous return (due to marked venous dilatation, as well as to decreased volume), (2) weaker cardiac contractions, and (3) a faster but weaker heart rate. These all lead to decreased cardiac output. Cardiac arrhythmias may occur. With an increasing loss of blood, there is less blood flow to the coronaries; hence, a relative state of myocardial weakness results. Even though the blood volume is markedly decreased, with myocardial failure the blood will not empty sufficiently into the four pulmonary veins, left atria, and left ventricle;
Auscultation of lungs. Moist rales.	it can dam up in the pulmonary capillary circuit, leading to an increased blood volume in the lungs. Hemorrhagic shock leads to constriction of the pulmonary artery and increased constriction of precapillary sphincters in the pulmonary blood vessels—which
PWP = 24.	leads to focal hemorrhages due to the damaging effect of increased pulmonary artery pressure on the precapillary sphincters. This, in turn, leads to increased interstitial plasma

151

Signs and symptoms (what?)	Physiological explanations (why?) and compensatory mechanisms
	in the pulmonary beds. An increasing PWP indicates a failing left ventricle.
Short of breath. Absence of breath sounds in right lower lobe.	Besides the decreased oxygen-carrying power of the blood, atelectatic changes may be occurring in the lungs. Decreased O_2, increased CO_2, and increased hydrogen ion concentration are all stimulants of respiration. The acidotic state continues and is reflected in the blood gases and pH of the blood. (Alkalosis sometimes develops early in shock due to compensatory hyperpnea.) A state of acidosis negates the effects of the catecholamines; hence, the peripheral blood vessels dilate markedly at this time. Less blood flow to the vasomotor center accentu-
CVP = 20 Cm. H2O.	ates the dilatation. A rising CVP indicates a failing right heart. Additional I.V. fluids, without strengthening the heart could drown him. The blood is very viscous, and is moving very slowly in the capillaries. Pooling, sludging, and disseminated intravascular clotting (D.I.C.) can occur at this time.
Respirations 40/min.	The increased respiratory rate will be followed by respiratory depression, unless the shock state is reversed with adequate treatment.
Sensorium dulled; listless and dizzy.	The sensorium is the best indication of adequacy of cerebral blood flow. Since blood-loss is continuing and compensatory mecha-
Stuporous; difficult to arouse.	nisms are waning, there is a decreased amount of oxygenated blood to the brain. The glucose supply to the brain has diminished. Since the functioning brain cells are dependent on carbohydrate metabolism, and since the metabolic process depends on oxygen, the brain metabolism is decreased.
BP = 80/30 M.A.P. = 47 mm. Hg. anuria persists.	At least 40 mm. Hg. pressure is required to convey blood to the brain. The systolic pressure is an important factor in the maintenance of cerebral blood flow. Therefore, a decrease in systolic pressure is accompanied by a decrease in the flow of blood to the brain. When the systolic pressure is 85 or below, and the signs and symptoms of shock are present, the loss of blood volume is at

Signs and symptoms (what?)	*Physiological explanations* (why?) *and compensatory mechanisms*
	least 40% or more. An acute hypovolemia exists.
Severe shock Approximately 45–50% loss of total blood volume BP = 68/0 M.A.P. = 23 mm. Hg.	A profound state of peripheral arteriolar dilatation exists, as indicated by the zero diastolic BP. Venous dilatation is evident. With decreased blood volume and dilated veins, the veins collapse under slight digital pressure.
Pulse 124/min., irregular, weak, barely perceptible.	The continued exposure of the heart to a high CO_2 tension causes a weakening of the heart beat and irregular rhythm. The amount of blood the myocardium receives for its functioning is dangerously reduced.
Unconscious.	Hypoxia of the brain cells develops to the extent that the brain cannot function normally; hence, unconsciousness develops.
Skin ashen gray and cold. Palms very pale, as well as soles of feet.	Due to a marked reduced hemoglobin; hence, decreased oxygen-carrying power.
Respirations 16 and decreasing.	This indicates depression of the respiratory center in the medulla oblongata. Any respiratory obstruction will cause respiratory acidosis.
Frank cyanosis of nail beds, lips, buccal mucosa and conjunctiva.	Cyanosis usually indicates the presence of excessive amounts of deoxygenated blood in the capillaries of the skin. The flow of blood within the capillaries is very sluggish at this time. Several factors determine the degree of cyanosis. These are

1. The quantity of deoxygenated hemoglobin in the arterial blood. Deoxygenated hemoglobin has a very intense, dark, bluish-red color. Frank cyanosis usually appears whenever the arterial blood contains more than 5 gm.% of deoxygenated hemoglobin. Very mild cyanosis appears when as little as 3 to 4 gm.% of deoxygenated hemoglobin is present.
2. The rate of blood flow through the skin. It is mainly the blood in the capillaries that determines the color of the skin. The dark bluish-red color of this blood is determined by two factors:

Signs and symptoms (what?)	Physiological explanations (why?) and compensatory mechanisms
	a. The concentration of deoxygenated hemoglobin in the arterial blood that enters the capillaries.
	b. The concentration of deoxygenation that occurs as the blood passes through the capillary bed.
	3. The pigmentation in the skin affects the degree to which cyanosis is visible. One cannot readily observe cyanosis in the darker Negro, however, cyanosis can be observed in the mucous membranes of the mouth, conjunctiva, palms, and soles.
	4. The thickness of the skin affects the blueness. For example, newborn babies have very thin skin; therefore, cyanosis can be detected rapidly, especially in the highly vascular parts of the body such as the heels.
Clammy skin (water, sodium and chloride loss through the pores of the skin).	One of the final signs of shock, clamminess indicates activation of sympathetic cholinergic fibers innervating the sweat glands. There is an acute deficit of vascular fluid, and an extensive deficit of sodium and chloride. Because the patient is anuric, sodium chloride and water leave via the skin.
Temperature decreasing, 96.	In severe shock, the thermoregulating mechanism is disturbed and the temperature decreases. Since heat is associated with the degree of metabolism, Mr. Kane's metabolism is very low.
Decreased breath sounds. Increasing rales.	Respiratory assistance and suctioning is certainly indicated. Atelectatic patches may be present at this time. When oliguria or anuria is due to poor renal perfusion as a result of general circulatory inadequacy, the patient is threatened with progressive deterioration of circulatory function unless corrective measures are taken promptly.
Kidney failure; anuria persists.	Often, anuria is attributed to kidney failure and believed to be the cause of the metabolic acidosis which dominates the terminal picture of fatal shock, when actually the anuria is only a reflection of inadequate circulation to the kidneys and to the body as a whole.

Signs and symptoms (what?)	Physiological explanations (why?) and compensatory mechanisms
	In such cases it is the inadequate perfusion of body tissues which produces the metabolic acidosis, and this metabolic deficiency in turn causes further derangements of cardiovascular function leading to progressive and even lethal circulatory failure.

Implications for Treatment of Patients in Hypovolemic Shock

The first step in treating the patient in hemorrhage is to identify the source of the bleeding and to take the necessary steps to stop it. This frequently requires surgical intervention. If the bleeding is external, pressure should be applied appropriately.

INTRAVENOUS SOLUTIONS

The choice of intravenous solutions should be based on the needs of the patient and on the physiologic role of the solution. Intravenous therapy for hemorrhagic shock is controversial. Following are some different viewpoints on this subject.

1. It is the general concensus that a judicious mixture of whole blood and crystalloid (electrolyte) solutions (such as Ringer's Lactate or Hartman's solution)* should be administered intravenously to the hemorrhaging patient. This provides for an effective balance of red blood cells, colloid (C.O.P.), and fluid, and electrolytes; which, in turn, provide for increased oxygen-carrying capacity and volume distribution between the three fluid compartments. Whole blood, alone, will not replenish the interstitial and intracellular compartments.

2. According to Moss, up to 75 per cent of the whole blood that has been lost can safely be replaced if sufficiently large volumes of crystalloid solutions are given. It is believed that the normal blood volume in the vascular compartment is maintained by moderate to marked expansion of the interstitial fluid. However, the limit for crystalloid replacement of whole blood should be based on the hematocrit

* About the same as the electrolyte concentration in the extracellular fluid.

155

level. If the hematocrit falls below 30 per cent, there will not be enough red blood cells to carry a sufficient amount of oxygen. Whole blood is indicated at this time.[1]

Since shock results in capillary wall weakness, capillary permeability will be increased. Therefore, the administration of colloid solutions would increase the colloid osmotic pressure in the interstitial compartment and hold volumes of fluid there. This, of course, would not benefit the circulating blood volume. The liver produces new plasma proteins, and, since plasma proteins also come from the plasma protein stores, then most of the plasma albumin deficit is repaired in 12–24 hours.

The danger of overtransfusing with colloids (such as plasma, albumin, and whole blood) is greater than transfusing with excess crystalloids, since colloids normally only occupy the vascular compartment.

OTHER SOLUTIONS: PRO AND CON

1. Plasma. Plasma carries the risk of viral hepatitis; therefore, its use should be limited.

2. Albumin. Albumin is considered an ideal volume replacement, as it increases the colloid osmotic pressure in the vascular compartment. It is a good substitute until whole blood is available.

3. Dextran. Dextran is a synthetic colloid plasma expander. Like protein (C.O.P.), dextran pulls fluid from the interstitial compartment into the vascular compartment, thus increasing the circulating blood volume. Dextran remains in the blood stream and does not pass into the interstitial compartment. When more than 1000 cc. of Dextran is used, an increased bleeding time may occur. Allergic reactions to it may also occur. In patients who have decreased renal tubular flow, dextran is contraindicated because it may cause obstruction of the renal tubules.

On the positive side, Dextran is favored in the postshock state to prevent the formation of platelet thrombi and to increase the flow in the capillaries.

4. Packed Cells. The plasma volume of packed cells is 50 per cent that of whole blood. Packed cells are advantageous in reducing the risk of blood-mismatching, allergic reactions, and hepatitis. They are also useful in maintaining the hematocrit.

One half and one fourth per cent Normal saline and 5 per cent

---

[1] G. Moss. "Fluid Distribution After Dilutional Hemoexpansion," *Surgical Forum* (1968), 27.

Glucose solutions should never be given in emergencies to hypovolemic patients, as they are hypotonic solutions and may lead to water-intoxication. (See p. 20 for review of isotonic, hypotonic, and hypertonic solutions.)

INDICATION FOR ANTIBIOTICS IN HYPOVOLEMIC SHOCK

When hypovolemia is severe, the tissues become progressively weaker. During the course of shock, besides the shift of blood from the peripheral blood vessels to the viscera, there is also a compensatory shunting of blood from the abdominal viscus to the major organs. This causes a relative degree of ischemia to the tissues of the gastrointestinal tract. Consequently, the weakness of these tissues is accentuated. With occlusion of the superior mesenteric artery, severe intestinal ischemia results, followed by sloughing of the intestinal musoca.

Studies have revealed that circulating endotoxins can be identified as early as five minutes after the occlusion of the superior mesenteric artery.[2] Weakness of the intestinal wall facilitates the exit of bacteria into the peritoneal cavity, leading to peritonitis. For this reason, antibiotics are justified in patients with hypovolemic shock.[3]

TREATMENT FOR RESPIRATORY DISTRESS SYNDROME

The following are indicated for the patient with respiratory distress:

1. An endotracheal tube to ensure patency of the upper respiratory tract. This facilitates suctioning as well as connection to a respirator.
2. Mechanical ventilation with positive end expiratory pressure (PEEP).
3. Frequent blood gases and blood pH determinations.
4. Albumin, intravenously, to increase the colloid osmotic pressure, thus pulling fluids from the pulmonary interstitial compartment into the blood.

[2] P. Cuevas and J. Fine. "Rout of Absorption of Endotoxin from the Intestine in Nonseptic Shock," *Journal of Reticuloenothelial Soc.* (1972), 535.
[3] Ronald Lee Nichols. "Antibiotics in Hypovolemic Shock," in *Treatment of Shock: Principles and Practices* (W. Schumer and L. Nyhus, eds.), Philadelphia: Lea and Febiger, 1974, pp. 168, 169.

5. Cardiotonic drugs to increase cardiac output, thus relieving the pressure of fluid in the pulmonary circulation.

6. The administration of oxygen.

Contraindications of the use of vasoconstrictors during hypovolemia

The administration of vasoconstrictor drugs during hypovolemia is contraindicated, as they would reduce the already depleted volume of plasma. By constricting the veins, the capillary pressure would be increased, thereby preventing the flow of fluid out of the capillaries and interstitial compartment.

External synchronized counterpulsation: treatment for the future?[4]

With the lower half of the body encased in an impervious plastic suit, pressure variations are produced by the rapid movement of water in and out of the suit. When negative and positive pressures are applied alternately, the venous return to the right heart is increased.

Nursing Care of Patients in Hemorrhagic Shock

Our steps must be guided by a clue, and the whole way from the very first perception of the senses must be laid out upon a sure plan.[5] As Beland has written:

"To justify a position among the professions, nursing must not only have some function which it can perform better than other professions, but it must be able to exercise independent judgment in the performance of these functions. Basic to sound judgment is knowledge." This knowledge *need not be unique* to the profession and may be derived from such disciplines as the biological, physical, and medical sciences as well as the humanities; however, it must be selected and organized in a way that is useful to the practice of the profession. Further, this knowledge should be selected and organized in terms of concepts and principles rather than by "rules of thumb."[6]

[4] Sheldon O. Burman and Decio O. Elias, "Mechanical and Circulatory Assistance in Shock," in *Treatment of Shock: Principles and Practices* (W. Schumer and L. Nyhus, eds.), Philadelphia: Lea and Febiger, 1974, pp. 173–182.
[5] Francis Bacon. "Preface to the Instauratio Magna."
[6] F. Abdellah, I. Beland, A. Martin and R. Matheny. *Patient-Centered Approaches to Nursing,* New York: Macmillan Publishing Company, Inc., 1960, p. 165.

The full-blown and easily recognized syndrome of shock is characterized by restlessness, anxiety, hypotension, pallor, cold clammy skin,
rapid thready pulse, and cyanosis of lips and nail beds. However, if
one is on the alert to identify the more subtle early signs of circulatory
inadequacy (characterized by a mild hypotension, tachycardia, or oliguria), the full-blown syndrome of shock, in many instances, need not
occur. In this respect, the nurse has an obligatory preventive role.

Primary interest should be centered on the effective perfusion
of blood to body tissues, rather than on the arterial blood pressure
level alone. Even if the blood pressure is within the patient's normal
range, marginal or inadequate circulation of blood should be suspected
if the following exist: apprehension, narrow pulse pressure, tachycardia,
clammy skin with poor color, or oliguria. It is hoped that the nurse
will realize that her responsibilities in the care of all patients center
in her observations of the whole patient, rather than on vital signs
alone, and that a blood pressure close to the patient's normal blood
pressure is, at the beginning of shock, an indication of his compensatory
mechanisms at work. The sooner the manifestations of impending
shock are detected and reported, the better chance the patient will
have for complete recovery.

As we proceed to discuss the objectives and principles of care,
keep the following four stages of shock in mind:

1. Initial stage. There is a decreased circulating blood volume,
   but not low enough to cause serious symptoms.
2. Compensatory stage. A further reduction of blood volume, but
   the blood pressure tends to stay within a normal range because
   of vasoconstriction. Blood flow to the skin and kidneys decreases. Blood flow to the central nervous system and the myocardium tends to be maintained. The blood reservoirs are decreased.
3. Progressive stage. Unfavorable changes become more and
   more apparent: falling blood pressure, increasing vasoconstriction, increased heart rate, and oliguria. In this progressive stage
   the compensatory mechanisms are unable to cope with the
   decreasing blood volume; therefore, the status quo is not maintained.
4. Irreversible stage. Treatment is no longer successful in saving
   the patient's life. Infused blood tends to remain in the dilated

capillary bed. There are a loss of arteriolar tonus and a myocardial depression.

The overall objectives and principles underlying the nursing care of any patient in hemorrhagic shock are the same. However, it must be remembered that different degrees of shock and variations of individual physiologic responses to shock necessitate "custom-fit" nursing care, so to speak, for the individual patient, or, if you prefer, "individualized" nursing care.

Continued hemorrhage implies
    Decreased blood volume
    Decreased venous return
    Decreased cardiac output
    Decreased blood pressure
    Decreased oxygen and nutrients to body tissues
    Decreased removal of cellular wastes
    Increased cellular anoxia (hypoxia)
    Decreased function of cells

"The inclusion of basic principles of nursing and beginning competence in the use of intellectual skills in applying nursing theory lays the groundwork for a continuing accretion of knowledge and competence."[7]
—*Martha E. Rogers*

Objectives, Principles, and Implications for Nursing Care

OBJECTIVE 1:   Provide for a continuous flow of blood to the brain. Facilitate the flow of blood to the brain.
PRINCIPLE 31:   The survival of brain cells is dependent on a continuous supply of oxygen and nutrients.
PRINCIPLE 32:   Increased specialization of a unit is accompanied by increased vulnerability of that unit.
PRINCIPLE 33:   The preservation of a vital part should have precedence over the preservation of less vital parts, even at the expense of the less vital parts.
PRINCIPLE 34:   Fluids and gases flow from greater to lesser points of pressure.

[7] Martha E. Rogers. *Educational Revolution in Nursing,* New York: Macmillan Publishing Co., Inc., 1961, p. 34.

Permanent brain damage can result within a few minutes if blood does not circulate to the brain in sufficient quantity. Other tissues, however, can be deprived of blood for a longer period of time without any untoward consequences.

NURSING CARE

Positioning of patient

The patient should be placed in a position that will provide for an adequate flow of blood *to* the brain, and *from* the brain back to the heart. The supine position is the position of choice to achieve this.* In cases of severe hemorrhage, this position can be modified to mobilize the blood from the legs, i.e., a supine position with the legs elevated on pillows to a 20 to 30 degree angle.

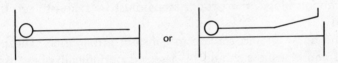

A Trendelenberg position (head down) should *not* be used! Although such a position facilitates the flow of blood to the brain, it *hinders* the return of venous blood from the brain back to the heart, thus the blood pools in the brain and hypoxia occurs there. At a Shock Unit in Los Angeles, doctors examined the hemodynamic effects of the head-down (Trendelenberg) position of shock patients. After a half hour, they found that the intra-arterial pressure and the cardiac output were decreased, rather than increased. When the patients were returned to the horizontal (supine) position, cardiac output improved.[8]

Other contraindications of the Trendelenberg position:

1. It hinders the flow of oxygenated blood from the pulmonary blood stream to the left atrium.
2. It causes the abdominal organs to push upward against the diaphragm, thus decreasing the area for pulmonary expansion, decreasing the effectiveness of the respiratory pump mechanism and therefore decreasing the volume of gaseous exchange of oxygen and carbon dioxide.

* If the patient has a skull or brain injury, he should be placed in a low Fowler's position to prevent excessive edema of the brain.
[8] Max Weil and Herbert Shubin. *Diagnosis and Treatment of Shock*, Baltimore: Williams and Wilkins Co., 1967, pp. 238–239.

Apprehension, dizziness, restlessness, and decreased levels of consciousness are all indications that the amount of blood flow to the brain is deficient. The brain, being most sensitive to the deleterious effects of a decreased blood supply, gives rise to symptoms that dominate the clinical picture. Acute hypoxia of the brain, therefore, produces impairment of judgment, motor incoordination, and a clinical picture which closely resembles that of acute alcoholism. When hypoxia is of long standing, the symptoms consist of fatigue, drowsiness, apathy, inattentiveness, and delayed reaction time simulating manifestations of severe fatigue. Unless blood is supplied to the brain, eventually the brain stem centers will be affected, and death resulting from respiratory failure will result, the gasping reflex persisting to the last.

Along with proper positioning, the patient needs blood. If blood is being administered, the rate should be increased. If the patient is not receiving blood, the proper steps must be taken to see that it is ordered.

The nurse should remain in constant attendance. The patient's level of consciousness should be assessed periodically, because this is an indication of whether the brain is receiving blood in sufficient quantity to sustain or to restore consciousness.

OBJECTIVE 2: Provide for adequate respirations.
PRINCIPLE 35: Oxygen is necessary to sustain life.
PRINCIPLE 36: The passage of oxygen from the atmosphere to the lungs and the passage of carbon dioxide from the blood stream to the atmosphere are dependent on an open airway.

Respirations, as with the pulse and blood pressure, should be checked every 15 minutes. Since the loss of blood implies a decreased oxygen- and carbon-dioxide-carrying power, the respiratory rate increases. The respiratory rate usually increases with the pulse rate, but not always in proportion. More commonly, the pulse increases out of proportion to the increase in respirations. However, if the airway is partially obstructed, the respiratory rate may increase out of proportion to the increase in the pulse rate.

The decreased oxygen content resulting from hemorrhage may be accentuated, and even complicated, by an obstructed airway. While it is obvious that a subnormal blood volume will increase the respiratory rate, it could be hazardous to assume that it is the only cause of an increased respiratory rate. If a decreased blood volume is the only reason for the increased respiratory rate, the respiratory rate will decrease with the replacement of blood. However, if the respiratory rate remains high, despite adequate blood replacement, airway obstruction should be suspected. Ignorance of this fact could lead to overtransfusion, which, in turn, could lead to pulmonary congestion and death. For this reason, it is imperative to be on the alert for any signs of respiratory obstruction.

Care should be taken that the patient's tongue does not relax back and shut off the air passage to his throat. If this occurs, the tongue should be pulled forward, and the patient should be placed on his side. Another factor that can cause obstruction of the air passages is secretions. Tracheobronchial secretions can occlude any part of the respiratory passages, including the nasal passages, pharynx, larynx, bronchi, bronchial tubes, and bronchioles. This can occur in any postoperative patient, because anesthetics and instruments used in administering anesthetics (such as the endotracheal tube) are irritating to the mucosal lining of the respiratory tree; hence, excess amounts of mucus are produced. Morphine and anesthetic agents dull the cough reflex and the ciliary motion, which further accentuates an underelimination of tracheobronchial secretions. Unless these secretions are removed, the amount of inspired oxygen and expired carbon dioxide will be reduced.

The increased respiratory rate of the patient in hemorrhagic shock may be caused by respiratory secretions that are blocking the air passages, as well as by the decreased blood volume. For this reason, it is always wise to have a suction machine readily available so it can be used when necessary. An obstructed airway leads to hypoventilation hypoxia, which in turn causes a marked decrease in the oxygen intake and carbon dioxide output. The arterial blood therefore will be (1) deficient in oxygen, and (2) saturated with carbon dioxide (hypercapnia).

Noisy breathing indicates the presence of respiratory secretions. The respirations should be observed for any wheezing, because wheezing occurs with bronchial obstruction from any cause. Also, if expiration is longer in duration than inspiration, bronchial obstruction is almost certain. Unless the respiratory sounds are audible to the ear, it is wise to use the stethoscope, applied to the upper midchest and the lower neck regions. Many times noisy or wheezing breathing cannot be detected with the ear, therefore it is preferable to use the stethoscope.

When the suction catheter is used, care should be taken to prevent irritation and trauma of the mucosal linings of the respiratory tract.

Irritation or trauma to this area could cause marked edema, which would only add insult to injury as far as respirations are concerned. If oronasal suctioning does not relieve the patient of his secretions, tracheal bronchial suctioning is indicated. It is well to have a tracheotomy tray in the patient's room, in case it is needed.

The administration of oxygen in the presence of a respiratory obstruction would be useless. Oxygen, however, can be useful if the increased respiratory rate is due solely to a low blood volume. The oxygen, administered by nasal catheter or by mask, would saturate the hemoglobin in the remaining red blood cells. There is, however, a marginal limit to which the hemoglobin can be saturated. If the lack of oxygen is due solely to the low blood volume, the best measure to decrease the respiratory rate would be to restore the blood volume, so that the capacity for carrying oxygen is increased.

OBJECTIVE 3: Support and maintain the compensatory mechanisms of the body, insofar as possible.
PRINCIPLE 26: Adaptation is basic to survival.
PRINCIPLE 37: Every living organism is provided with a means to protect itself.
PRINCIPLE 38: The length of time and the degree to which self-protection can be maintained are variable in different individuals.
OBJECTIVE 4: Decrease the patient's metabolic needs.
PRINCIPLE 39: There is a relative proportion between cellular activity and cellular requirements for oxygen and nutrients (blood).
    a. Increased cellular activity (metabolism) implies an increased need for oxygen and nutrients.
    b. Decreased cellular activity implies a decreased need for oxygen and nutrients.

The maintenance of an adequate circulation of blood is dependent on three mechanisms: (1) blood volume, (2) cardiac muscle pump mechanism, and (3) vascular resistance. It has been amply demonstrated that, with the deficiency or failure of any one of these mechanisms, the other two compensate for the deficiency. In this instance, the loss of blood is compensated for by an increased heart rate and peripheral vascular constriction.

Always remember, one of the paramount responsibilities of the nurse is to support the defensive compensatory mechanisms of the body. Failure to understand the actions of these mechanisms might lead the nurse to counter the life-saving effects provided by nature.

A main compensatory mechanism at work within the body of a patient suffering from hemorrhagic shock is the result of sympathetic nervous system and adrenal medullary stimulation. This sympathoadrenal medullary mechanism is responsible for shifting blood from peripheral vessels of tissues needing it less to internal visceral vessels whose tissues need it most. This, as has been mentioned, is accomplished by the vasoconstriction action of norepinephrine. As a result of this vasoconstriction, the blood pressure may remain within a normal range for the patient for a short period of time, despite his loss of blood. It should be remembered, however, that a near-normal blood pressure in the presence of cool, pale skin is an indication of these compensatory mechanisms at work. Failure to appreciate this might lead the nurse to thwart this compensation. The nonshivering patient should be kept cool. Heat, in any form, if applied to the patient, would dilate the peripheral blood vessels of the skin, thus counteracting the effects of vasoconstriction. The blood, which is needed so desperately by the vital organs, would be drawn back into the peripheral vessels of the skin. Only if the patient is shivering should external heat be applied, and in that case the patient should be covered just enough to stop the shivering. Shivering is caused by rhythmic muscle contraction; therefore, the metabolic effects of shivering resemble those of light exercise. The oxygen consumption rate can increase to 3.7 times basal in 15 minutes with shivering.

Not only will heat cause peripheral vasodilatation, but it will also raise the body temperature. An elevation of body temperature of 1 degree Centigrade will increase the body metabolism by 7 per cent. Increased metabolism, in turn, implies an increased need for oxygen and an increased production of carbon dioxide, both of which place additional burdens on the already overtaxed heart and respiratory system. Heat also leads to sweating, which, through the loss of sodium chloride and water, decreases the volume of circulating fluid even further. In a word, the application of heat to the patient in hemorrhagic shock would deepen his shock state.

If, for any reason, the body temperature is elevated to 102° F or over, it should be combated by the use of sponging or fans. Although moderate elevation of metabolism is harmless in the presence of a normal circulation, it may prove hazardous when the blood supply to the tissues is inadequate.

Blankets and other heat-retaining or -producing elements should

be *removed* from the patient. The patient should be covered just sufficiently to prevent chilling and shivering.

Replacement of blood volume will relieve the stress on the compensatory mechanisms.

OBJECTIVE 5:   Provide for the judicious relief of pain.

PRINCIPLE 40:   Pain intensifies the degree of shock.

PRINCIPLE 41:   Anything that can affect man may influence his tolerance to pain.

The following factors are among the more important of those
that influence tolerance to pain:

Age—the very young and the very old have a relatively high
tolerance.

Sex—a greater tolerance in females.

Fatigue, fear, noise, excessive heat, cold and light lower the tolerance.

Nervousness and anxiety lower the tolerance to pain.

Endocrine factors, for example, hyperthyroidism, the climacteric,
and adrenal insufficiency lower the tolerance to pain.

Effects of drugs modify the activity of the central nervous system.

Conditions such as anemia, malnutrition, hypoproteinemia, and
lowered vitality lower the tolerance to pain, also.

Pain is both a symptom and a sensation. As a symptom, pain is
a warning of danger. When pain is severe, the use of narcotics should
be judicious. Due consideration and precautions should be exercised,
because any of the following factors could cause the patient to respond
excessively to narcotics: shock, renal impairment, hepatic impairment,
decreased pulmonary function, and advanced age.

One knows that most drugs taken into the body—whether via
the oral, subcutaneous, intramuscular, or intravenous route—are absorbed, eventually, into the blood stream. (Intravenous, of course, implies direct admission into the blood stream.) The healthy individual
absorbs drugs into a blood stream greater in quantity than that of a
patient in hemorrhagic shock. Therefore, in hemorrhagic shock, the
decreased blood volume predisposes to a delay in the absorption of
drugs. With the improvement of the circulatory status through the
replacement of blood, or other fluids, there may be a sudden and
intense narcotic effect. The physician usually takes these factors into

consideration when he orders the dosage of drugs and the time interval for administration.

The nurse must be on the alert for any signs or symptoms of toxicity due to drugs; this includes all other drugs that the patient may be receiving. The effects of drugs that lower arterial blood pressure, pulse rate, and respiratory rate must be taken carefully into account.

The unconscious patient may react to pain without feeling pain in any specific area. His reaction is usually caused by a dull, generalized discomfort and may include groaning, mild restlessness, and/or defensive thrashing movements in bed. Simple, involuntary, or unconditioned reactions to pain can occur at any level of the peripheral afferent nerve transmission system and are not necessarily impaired by a state of unconsciousness.

On the other hand, sensation of pain impulses is dependent on a state of consciousness and the integrity of the thalamocortical system of the brain. This might be explained further. In hemorrhagic shock, a state of unconsciousness is due to a decreased amount of blood to the brain. As a result, the brain tissues are deprived of oxygen and nutrients that are vitally necessary for proper brain functioning. The central motor and sensory areas, deprived of sufficient blood, cannot carry on their normal functions of receiving sensory impulses and transmitting motor impulses. Some patients in moderate or severe stages of shock, therefore, might not require medication for the relief of pain, simply because they lack the sensation of pain. Any degree of pain, however, in the presence of hemorrhage, burns, or severe trauma increases the liability of shock and can aggravate the severity of shock through its paralyzing effects on the vasomotor center which would lead to massive vasodilatation. Therefore, by alleviating the patient's pain, more severe insulting degrees of shock can often be avoided.

When a narcotic is required, a small intravenous dose is likely to be as effective as a larger dose given subcutaneously. A small dose early will do more than a large dose later. Delay in administering analgesics decreases their effectiveness. It must be remembered that narcotic poisoning can result from multiple subcutaneous doses of morphine, since the narcotic may remain unabsorbed until the blood volume and flow are restored by transfusion.

While it is important for the nurse to know when to withhold narcotics from patients, it is equally important that she knows when

167

not to withhold them. Narcotics that should be given are withheld in far too many instances.

In the preceding paragraphs, by no means are "always" and "never" implied. The final decision must be based upon the condition and needs of the individual patient. Withholding a narcotic from a patient who needs it on the basis of an unjustified fear that "the patient might become addicted" is foolish.

OBJECTIVE 6:   Provide for adequate circulation of blood to all body areas.
SUBOBJECTIVES: a. Provide for adequate venous return.
   b. Provide for adequate cardiac output.
   c. Provide for adequate nutrition and oxygenation of all body cells.
   d. Provide for adequate removal of cellular wastes.
PRINCIPLE 16:   The heart can eject into the arterial circuit only that amount of blood it receives from the venous circuit.
PRINCIPLE 42:   The life and proper functioning of all body tissues depend on an adequate supply of blood.

It is obvious that the primary need of the patient in hemorrhagic shock is the replacement of his circulating fluid. A delay in restoring adequate circulation may prove fatal through the serious renal and cardiovascular complications that may ensue. If the decreased blood pressure is due to hypovolemia alone, the arterial blood pressure will respond quickly to rapid blood volume replacement. If, however, the arterial blood pressure does not increase after 500 to 750 ml. of blood has been given, the cause of the decreased blood pressure is probably other than hypovolemia.

If the patient is receiving blood, the nurse should increase the rate of flow. While it is not the nurse's prerogative to administer blood, or any solution intravenously, it is, nevertheless, vital that she recognizes the patient's need for intravenous replacement of fluid, and takes the necessary steps toward seeing that he receives it. This includes seeing that the physician is notified for the final decision and having the necessary solutions and supplies readily available. It is always best that the nurse remain at the patient's bedside, because only the professional nurse is equipped with those judgments needed in emergency situations. Hospitals usually have their own signaling devices to be used for emergency situations, be it an intercom system, buzzer, or light system.

In the event that whole blood is used, no matter how crucial the patient's need for blood, the blood typing, cross match, and Rh factor should always be checked against the patient's laboratory record to ensure his receiving the correct blood. If blood of a different type is administered, agglutination (clumping) of the red blood cells will occur, which can lead to renal failure and death.

At the onset of shock, the only clue may be apprehension of the patient. This is a sufficient indication for the nurse to remain with the patient and to check his blood pressure and other vital signs at least every 15 minutes. A written record of these vital signs should be kept at the patient's bedside. At this time, the nurse should also check for other signs and symptoms; this includes taking note of his skin color and temperature, restlessness, dizziness, and so forth.

Care should be taken that the patient isn't overtransfused with fluids. (This is another indication for keeping a close check on his blood pressure.) While the young adult can tolerate some excess of circulating fluid, the very young and the elderly cannot. The danger is, of course, circulatory overload which could lead to acute pulmonary edema and death from suffocation. For this reason, the nurse should know the patient's normal blood pressure, if this is at all possible. Knowing this, she can adjust the rate of flow of intravenous solutions accordingly, i.e., to slow the rate if the blood pressure approaches within 10 degrees of the patient's normal blood pressure. The normal blood pressure should be written at the top of the record slip and kept at the bedside, so that others in attendance may use it as a criterion. Unless the patient was admitted as an emergency, it is usually possible to find his normal blood pressure reading on his chart. It cannot be emphasized too strongly, that when the patient's normal blood pressure reading is available, it should be known by the nurse. Assumptions and guesses about the patient's normal blood pressure are highly out of order. What is a normal blood pressure for one person might be entirely different from the normal blood pressure of another. The hundred plus the age dictum is completely unscientific.

In known cases of hemorrhage, a systolic blood pressure below the patient's normal systolic pressure is indicative of a decreased blood volume. A diastolic pressure above the patient's normal diastolic would indicate increased peripheral resistance, which is a direct compensatory effect of sympathoadrenal medullary vasoconstriction action. A decline of the diastolic pressure is indicative of decreased peripheral resistance; hence, we would know that compensatory vasoconstriction is being replaced by vasodilation—an indication that the compensatory mechanisms no longer can compensate for the loss of blood. If the diastolic pressure falls to zero, it is a clear indication of a total lack of arteriolar resistance and that massive vasodilatation exists.

Source of bleeding

After the patient has been placed in a supine position and is receiving intravenous fluid, the source and nature of the bleeding should be determined. The color and rate of flow should be noted. Arterial blood is bright red and flows rapidly in spurts. Venous blood is dark red and oozes. If the bleeding is not external, it must be internal. If there is arterial bleeding from a limb, a tourniquet should be applied above the area of bleeding. If there is venous bleeding from a limb, a tourniquet should be applied below the area of bleeding. If the bleeding can be controlled with a pressure dressing, it should be used in preference to the tourniquet, because there is a certain element of danger in the use of tourniquets. A tourniquet should never be left on longer than necessary. If used, the tourniquet should be loosened at hourly intervals, in order to permit blood to flow to points below the bleeding area. Unless this is done, the tissues below the tourniquet would be deprived of blood; therefore, gangrene would set in.

The most obvious area to observe after any operation is the incisional area, or the pertinent body orifice, or both. Patients with gastric ulcers and esophageal varices may be bleeding internally and may or may not have hematemesis. Patients with known pulmonary disease may have a slow, oozing pulmonary hemorrhage with or without hemoptysis. And of course, any operation is accompanied by possible internal bleeding.

"Reinforcement" of dressings means to "add to" the original dressing. In cases of minimal incisional bleeding, it is often necessary to add a dressing. However, if the bleeding does not cease, the surgeon should be notified immediately. It is not excusable to add dressing after dressing after dressing. Unless the bleeding is checked (it is sometimes necessary to take the patient back to the operating room to tie off a bleeder) and blood replacement is made, the amount of blood lost into these dressings could prove fatal for the patient. In her reporting and recording, it is wise for the nurse to mention the type of dressing and the size of the bloody area on it. It is not sufficient to use terms such as "small," "moderate," or "large" amount of "drainage" on dressing. These words mean different things to different people.

More specific statements are necessary, such as "bright bloody drainage the size of a half-dollar on 4- × -4 dressing," or perhaps "bright bloody drainage the size of a half-dollar on ABD dressing." Even though the size of the drainage area might be the same on both types of dressings, it is obvious that the ABD dressing is thicker and can absorb a greater quantity of blood than the 4- × -4. If possible, a ruler should be used to measure the diameter of the bloody area. If a ruler is not available, comparisons familiar to all should be employed, i.e., the size of a dime, a quarter, half-dollar. If the blood is on the patient's clothing, that part of the clothing involved should be mentioned by the nurse, as some articles of clothing absorb more blood than other articles. For example, a sweater absorbs more blood than a shirt.

Thirst
The patient who has lost blood will complain of thirst, if he is conscious. It has been explained that fluid leaves the interstitial compartment and enters the vascular compartment to increase the volume of circulating fluid. Thirst, therefore, usually will be accompanied by other signs of dehydration. In the absence of nausea and vomiting or any gastrointestinal operation, it is usually permissible to give oral fluids if the patient is conscious and able to swallow. The patient's head, however, should not be raised. It should remain flat for obvious circulatory reasons. He should be instructed to turn his head to the side; then water, through a straw, can be given. There is much less possibility of aspirating if the head is turned to the side. Anesthetics and morphine slow the reflex action of the epiglottis. Therefore, it is wise to tell the patient to dry-swallow, before giving oral fluids. If he can do this, it is best to give him a sip of water to see how he handles it. Fluids given to the patient who has a slow reflex action of the epiglottis can lead to aspiration of the fluid into the respiratory tract which could lead to aspiration pneumonia. Elderly patients are more susceptible to pneumonia, because of their slower epiglottis reflex, and also because of limited expansion of the rib cage and poorer aeration of the lungs.

The pulse
The blood pressure is related inversely to the heart rate. A decreased blood pressure therefore will be accompanied by an increased heart rate, which is detectable in an arterial pulse. The pulse should be checked at frequent intervals, as well as the blood pressure. Check-

ing of the pulse is a very important measure and should never be regarded as "routine." Because the pulse beat reflects the heart beat, the rhythm of the heart often can be detected by the pulse. Besides the rate of the pulse being counted, it is equally important to note the quality of the pulse. Is it a full pulse (also referred to as a large, or bounding pulse), or is it a small, weak, or even flickering pulse? Is it perceptible or imperceptible? Is the rhythm regular or irregular? If it is irregular, is it a regular irregularity?

If the radial pulse cannot be detected, the pulse may be detectable in the temporal, facial, carotid, or femoral regions. If the radial pulse is irregular, it is wise to check the apical pulse simultaneously. For accuracy, this is better done by two persons—one counting the radial pulse, and the other, with a stethoscope, listening to and counting the heart sounds at its apex. The difference between the apical and the radial counts is known as the pulse deficit.

The pulse of a hemorrhaging patient is always rapid. The strength of the pulse usually wanes as the blood loss continues or is not replaced. On the other hand, the pulse becomes stronger and slower when the blood volume is increased.

OBJECTIVE 7: Relieve patient's apprehension.
PRINCIPLE 43: When physiological needs are threatening to a person's life, we reassure him mainly by what we *do* for him, rather than by what we *say* to him.

The principle implies the nursing course. However, it should be mentioned that a soft tone of voice, touch, and noiseless movements do much to decrease patients' psychological stress and apprehension.

The nurse must assess the probable cause of his apprehension, i.e., does it have a psychological or physiological basis? In all probability, Mr. Kane's apprehension is due to the physiological deficit of decreased blood to his brain. This leads directly to restlessness and apprehension which can only be relieved by intelligent and purposeful nursing actions.

Hypovolemic Shock Due To Plasma Loss

Certain conditions in which large amounts of plasma are lost can also lead to hypovolemic shock. Some of these are as follows.

SEVERE VENOUS OBSTRUCTION

An obstruction (such as phlebothrombosis) occurring in a major vein causes the capillary pressure distal to the obstruction to increase to the extent that large quantities of plasma fluid leak into the interstitial compartment. (An increased venous resistance leads to an increased capillary pressure.) As a consequence, large quantities of edema fluid accumulate in the interstitial compartment, and the circulating blood volume in the vascular compartment decreases.

Venous obstruction often occurs late in pregnancy. This is called "the supine hypotensive syndrome." This syndrome may occur when the pregnant woman assumes a supine position; a position in which the patient is usually placed by nurses and doctors. Within three to seven minutes in this position, a rapid weak pulse, cardiac palpitations, respiratory distress, decreased blood pressure, and diaphoresis may develop. If sufficiently severe, the patient may become unconscious. The cause of this is due to pressure of the gravid uterus on the inferior vena cava. According to Clausen, the treatment of this syndrome is simple; namely, "turn the patient on her side, or manually displace the uterus off of the inferior vena cava. Either action permits blood to flow freely through the inferior vena cava to the upper portion of the body."[9]

Shock resulting from this syndrome is obviously due to a decreased return of venous blood to the right heart; consequently, decreased

[9] Joy Clausen. "Hypotension: A Cause to Remember," *Nursing '72,* 2 (May 1972), 535.

Figure 18. *Increased venous resistance and the displacement of plasma from the intravascular compartment into the interstitial compartment. A decreased circulating blood volume and edema result.*

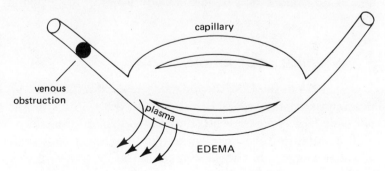

cardiac output results. To treat this patient with intravenous fluids and plasma expanders, or cardiotonic drugs, and so on is certainly *not* indicated, as a decreased blood volume and cardiac failure are not the cause of this type of shock.

THE NEPHROTIC SYNDROME

In the nephrotic syndrome, large amounts of protein are lost in the urine, so that normal plasma protein concentration cannot be maintained. As a result of this protein loss, the colloid osmotic pressure is decreased; hence, much of the fluid in the interstitial compartment remains there because the decreased colloid osmotic pressure in the vascular compartment cannot pull it into the vascular compartment. Edema results.

NUTRITIONAL HYPOVOLEMIA

Starvation can reduce the plasma proteins to such a low level that shock ensues. Because the decreased colloid osmotic pressure cannot pull fluids from the interstitial compartment into the vascular compartment, and the hydrostatic pressure at the arteriolar end of the capillaries exceeds the colloid osmotic pressure at the venous end, more fluid enters the interstitial compartment than leaves it. Severe edema and bloating result.

Any diet which is deficient in protein foods will lead to a relative state of hypoproteinemia. The mechanism is the same as in the nephrotic syndrome, i.e., decreased colloid osmotic pressure leading to edema. The basis of many of the present weight-loss programs is a high protein intake. Increased proteins mobilize increased amounts of fluid from the interstitial compartment. Considering that a pint of fluid is equivalent to a pound of body weight, many pounds can be lost.

INTESTINAL OBSTRUCTION

In 1974 in the U.S., the mortality rate from intestinal obstruction was approximately 10 per cent. In the early 1900s it was over 50 per cent. The decrease is attributed to gastrointestinal decompression with nasogastric tubes, and so on, fluid and electrolyte replacement, antibiotics, and better surgical techniques.

174

Intestinal obstructions occurring any place in the small or large intestine can lead to severe hypovolemia, due to the loss of excessive fluid and electrolytes into the lumen of the intestine. Some examples of bowel obstruction are adhesive bands, groin hernia, tumors, volvulus, intussusception, and so forth. In children, hernias are the most common cause.

Pathophysiology

The pathophysiology of intestinal obstructions is inclusive of the following:

1. Decreased insorption (absorption) from the intestinal lumen into the bowel.
2. Increased exorption, or secretion, from the intestinal blood stream into the lumen, which leads to fluid-loss. As the pressure in the lumen increases, secretion of fluid into the lumen increases. Consequently, fluid-loss and distention occur. The loss of potassium is usually three to six times more than normal in the obstructed intestine.

As a result, fluid accumulates in the lumen of the obstructed intestine, increasing the distention of that part. Increasing intraluminal pressure compresses the blood vessels in the intestinal tissue, leading to an impairment of its circulation with a subsequent weakness of the tissue. Therefore, fluids and electrolytes leak into the intestinal walls. Peritoneal fluid results from local serosal transudation of fluid.

In pyloric obstruction, metabolic alkalosis will result from loss of potassium chloride and hydrochloric acid from the stomach. Since potassium and chloride have been lost, treatment indicates a replacement of these two electrolytes.

If the obstruction is lower, i.e., in the upper small bowel, metabolic acidosis will occur, as bile and pancreatic secretion will be lost.

Distention can also be caused by intestinal gas. Increased motility of the proximal bowel with violent peristalsis will lead to edema of the bowel. Increased intraluminal pressure of the bowel causes lymphatic and capillary stasis. The venous drainage can thus be impaired. If the pressure rises to greater limits (above 90 mm. Hg.), the arterial flow will be occluded. The small bowel will burst if the intraluminal pressure gets as high as 120 to 230 mm. Hg. pressure.

When the contents within the bowel are stagnant, an increase in the number of bacteria occurs there. An increased intraluminal

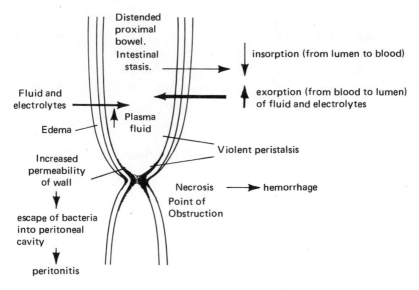

Figure 19. *Pathophysiological implications of bowel obstruction.*

pressure causes a decreased blood supply to that part of the intestine; therefore, ischemia, and subsequent necrosis of the bowel wall develops. Intestinal contents then escape into the peritoneal cavity and cause peritonitis.

Interference with the mesenteric blood supply is the most serious complication of bowel obstruction. This occurs secondary to the adhesive bands of the intestine, or strangulated hernia, volvulus, and so on, which decrease the blood flow through the mesenteric arteries; hence, weakness of the respective tissues occurs.

The loss of fluid and electrolytes depends on:

1. The degree of venous congestion (increased venous resistance leads to increased capillary pressure).
2. Amount of edema in the wall of the intestine.
3. Peritoneal transudation.
4. How long the obstruction has existed.
5. The degree of vomiting or gastrointestinal suction.

The results of intestinal obstruction are (1) hemoconcentration, because of the loss of plasma fluid into the lumen of the intestine, (2) decreased blood volume, (3) decreased urine output (due to renal insufficiency), and, unless treated immediately, ultimately, death.

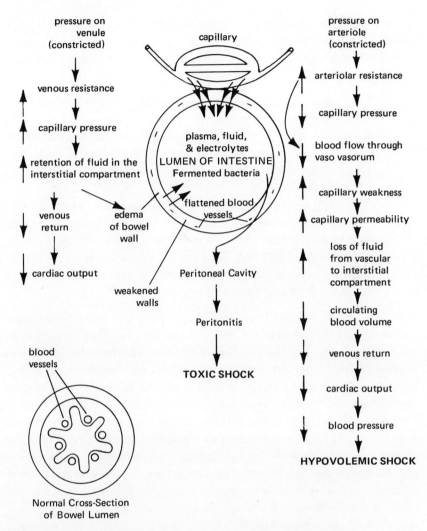

Figure 20. *Bowel obstruction: abnormal capillary dynamics leading to hypovolemic shock and toxic shock.*

Burn Shock

Burn shock is another example of hypovolemic shock. It is sometimes referred to as electrolyte shock or plasma loss shock. (Other conditions producing electrolyte shock are intestinal obstruction, fistulas, and severe diarrhea.) Burns can be caused by the exposure of the body to fire, a very high temperature of dry or moist heat, electricity, x-ray, radium, or corrosive chemicals. The prognosis of the patient depends more on the extent of the burn than on its depth. Burns are classified as follows:

1. First degree burn. Outer layer of skin is pink to slight red with blister formation. Painful.
2. Second degree burn. Skin is mottled red to deep pink, moist. Formation of blisters or blebs beneath the upper layer of skin. Deep layers are not destroyed. Most painful of the three types of burns.
3. Third degree burn. Skin is white or charred. Destruction of superficial, subcutaneous, and muscle tissue. Little to no pain due to destruction of nerve endings. All layers of the skin are destroyed, making regeneration impossible. Scar tissue formation, or need of skin graft. Nerves, muscles, and bone may be injured and sometimes destroyed.

Burn shock results from the loss of fluid and electrolytes from all three fluid compartments; plasma from the vascular compartment, sodium from the vascular and interstitial compartments (ECF), and potassium from the intracellular compartment. Primarily, however, burn shock is caused by the rapid shift of plasma fluid from the vascular compartment, across the heat-damaged capillaries, into the interstitial compartment and/or to the surface of the burned area. Plasma loss is in direct relation to the extent of the area burned. The transfer of plasma from the vascular compartment results in local tissue edema and weeping. As was stated, the loss is mainly plasma fluid rather than whole blood. However, in deep extensive burns, the red cell mass is usually lowered because of (1) hemolysis due to heat from the burn, (2) depression of red cell formation, (3) edema of the wound, and (4) altered iron and globin metabolism. (Damaged red blood cells within the damaged capillaries of the burned area may sludge which could lead to thrombosis.)

The loss of plasma fluid begins almost immediately after injury and reaches a peak within the first few hours. Burn shock, therefore, is mainly a problem of the first 24 to 36 hours after injury, and, if correct treatment and nursing care are instituted immediately, it is rarely a problem after 48 hours.

Burn shock is characterized by the following physiological alterations.

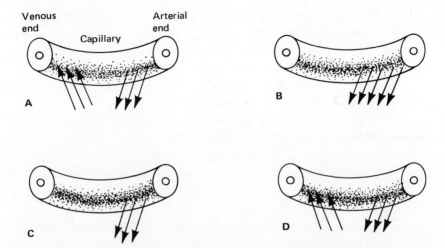

Figure 21. *Normal and abnormal transfer of fluid across the capillary membrane.*
    *A. Normal transfer of fluid out of and into the capillary. An
equilibrium between 1 and 2.*
    *B. Immediately after burn or injury. A marked disequilibrium. Fluid
leaves capillary but no fluid enters. Implications: (1) decreased blood volume,
and (2) increased edema formation. As many as 10 liters or more of plasmalike
fluid may accumulate in the tissues and therefore be unavailable to the
circulatory system.*
    C. Six to twelve hours after injury. Fluid loss declines.
    *D. After 24 hours. Equilibrium re-established. Implications: (1)
increasing blood volume, and (2) decreasing tissue edema. The critical period
of shock is over.*

1. Reduced blood volume, due to the extravasation of plasma
fluid into the interstitial compartment and to the surface of the burn.

    a. Increased arteriolar dilatation in the burn area* results in in-
creased capillary pressure leading to excessive plasma fluid-
loss from the vascular compartment into the interstitial compartment, thus raising the oncotic pressure in the interstitial
compartment.

    b. Damage to capillaries leads to increased capillary permeability
with the resultant loss of more fluids from the vascular compartment.

* In burn shock, there is a loss of peripheral resistance only at the site(s) of the burn
injury. Unaffected areas of the body respond with compensatory vasoconstriction which
maintains coronary perfusion and BP

2. Hemoconcentration (initially, there is an increased hematocrit), i.e., the red blood cell count and the hemoglobin are high in relation to the circulating blood plasma. A high blood viscosity results with an increasing predisposition to blood-clot formation.

3. Injured tissue cells since potassium leaves the injured cells, and sodium and water enter, causing cellular edema.

4. In large burn areas, increased metabolic rate may be as much as four to eight times normal. This is followed by marked heat-loss from the burn area. If the area burned is large, excessive heat will be lost from the body. Efforts are usually taken to prevent heat-loss by increasing the environmental temperature and humidity, and by the application of wet dressings.

5. Cardiac output ultimately decreases, owing to a decreased venous return.

6. Anemia, e.g., in large deep burns, up to 5 per cent of the red blood cells are immediately destroyed. Severe anemia usually occurs about a week following a large burn.

7. Respiratory complications, e.g., if the burn is due to steam, the lower respiratory tract may be injured. Inhalation of noxious gases and acids may cause necrosis of the alveolar membranes, edema, and infection.

8. Ileus of the gastrointestinal tract usually results from major burns. Patients usually complain of thirst. If they were to be given water to drink, acute gastric dilatation could occur. This could result in decreased respiratory efficiency, vomiting, and aspiration.

Curling's ulcer: upper gastrointestinal hemorrhage may occur seven to ten days postburn, and is usually in the stomach and/or duodenum. Epigastric pain and tenderness may be present. Conservative managment of nasogastric suction, antacids, and antispasmodics is usually followed. It is thought that Curling's ulcer is due to a profound stress reaction inclusive of an increase in histamine, adrenal cortical hormones, impaired blood flow due to increased sympathetic stimulation which constricts the blood vessels of the gastrointestinal tract, and poor cell-nutrition of the stomach and duodenum.

9. A decreased immune response. This may be decreased by intravenous hyperalimentation.

10. Renal failure may occur from circulatory changes associated with decreased blood volume, or from the effects of deep burns on the erythrocytes and myoglobin. An intense sympathetic nervous sys-

tem reaction leads to a decreased flow of blood through constricted renal blood vessels.

11. Infection may occur, due to the loss of skin—the first line of defense. Also, organisms grow best in a warm, moist, proteinous media. Should the infection reach the blood stream, a septicemia would, in all probability, occur. Rapid removal of dead tissue is indicated to attempt to prevent septicemia (toxic shock).

Burned patients are rarely unconscious. A severely burned person is alert and active, which contrasts sharply to some of the other shock patients. Decreased flow of blood to the brain of the burn patient, and decreased blood pressure is a late sign of burn shock.

CAPILLARY PERMEABILITY AND FLUID LOSS

Either the capillaries within the burned area are totally destroyed, or they are damaged to the extent that their walls become extremely fragile. Extensive capillary fragility results in extensive capillary permeability, which, in turn, results in the loss of large amounts of plasma proteins, water, and sodium to the interstitial compartment, and/or to the surface of the wound. If the burn is deep, the plasma accumulates in the interstitial compartment. If the burn is superficial, the plasma is lost to the surface. Because of the loss of plasma proteins from the vascular compartment, the capillary colloid osmotic pressure (oncotic pressure) is greatly diminished; therefore, the hydrostatic pressure at the arterial end of the capillary meets with little opposition from the decreased C.O.P. at the venous end. As a consequence, more fluid enters the interstitial compartment than leaves it. This shift of fluid, if untreated, will lead to marked hypovolemia, shock, and death.

STRESS REACTION

In response to extensive burns, a marked stress reaction occurs within the body. This stress reaction is a generalized systemic response, just as in hemorrhagic shock. The pituitary-adrenal cortical axis and the sympathoadrenal medullary mechanisms are stimulated. As a result, large amounts of aldosterone from the adrenal cortex act to conserve sodium, and hence water, in the body in an effort to raise the blood volume and the blood pressure. Copious amounts of norepinephrine from both the sympathetic nervous system and the adrenal medullae cause a generalized vasoconstriction, also for the purpose of elevating the blood pressure in an effort to sustain life. With renal arteriolar constriction resulting from the effects of norepinephrine, the glomerular filtrate pressure is decreased, hence oliguria or anuria may result, and the wastes ordinarily removed by the kidneys will remain in the blood stream.

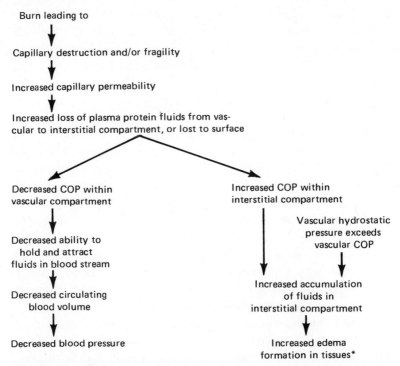

* Wound edema progresses during the acute phase. As much as 10 liters or more of plasmalike fluid may accumulate in the tissues and, therefore, be unavailable to the circulatory system.

Peripheral resistance is one of the factors determining the blood pressure; therefore, an increased peripheral resistance resulting from extensive vasoconstriction causes an increased blood pressure. The hypovolemia caused by the loss of plasma proteins, sodium, and water into the interstitial compartment may reach a critically low level, but because of the increased peripheral resistance (caused by the highly viscous blood) and the increased vasoconstriction, the blood pressure would not decline proportionately. Hence the recognition of shock might be delayed, and the treatment to correct the hypovolemic state might also be delayed until it is too late.

THE METABOLIC COURSE

The metabolic course of a patient with a severe 25 to 50 per cent surface area burn will follow four phases, unless the patient dies of shock in the first phase. While we are concerned primarily with the first phase, the other three phases will be mentioned at this time also, because the patient is never really out of danger of shock until a positive nitrogen balance has been re-established.

The four phases of the metabolic course

1. Shock, due to hypovolemia, is produced by:
   a. Loss of plasma proteins, water, and sodium from the damaged capillaries of the vascular compartment into the interstitial compartment, leading to
   b. Expansion of the interstitial compartment, edema formation. Ten to fifteen liters of high-electrolyte, plasmalike fluid collects as edema.
   c. Loss of potassium from the intracellular compartment. The potassium is replaced by sodium, therefore, normal cellular function is impaired.
   d. Renal insufficiency, due to renal arteriolar constriction and the retention of sodium and water. If urine is being produced, there will be a large loss of potassium in it.

   During this period there is almost total starvation of the patient, except for the small amount of dextrose he may be receiving intravenously.
2. Major adjustments begin two to three days after the burn, if the patient is responding adequately to treatment.
   a. Repair of capillary membranes. Abnormal seepage stops and the edema fluid is absorbed back into the vascular compartment (this includes plasma proteins, sodium, and water). With the shift of plasma back into the vascular compartment, the colloid osmotic pressure in the vascular compartment increases; thus more fluid from the interstitial compartment is drawn into the blood stream by osmosis. The restoration of a more normal colloid osmotic pressure in

183

the capillary blood stream counterbalances the hydrostatic pressure in the capillaries and thus stops the main mechanism that had contributed to edema formation. The shift of this fluid back into the circulatory stream endangers the patient, because overloading of the blood stream with subsequent hypervolemia may occur. Renal excretion in excess of 100 ml. per hour indicates the need for caution in the rate and amount of fluid given the patient parenterally. Normal urinary output ranges from 1000 to 1800 ml. per day (24-hour period). If we use as an average 1500 ml. per 24 hours, the hourly renal output would be 62.5 ml., or 1 ml. (15 gtt) per minute. In health, the kidneys of the normal, healthy individual must remove 35 gm. of solid material, or waste matter, from the blood each day.

    b. Increased urinary output. Sodium diuresis occurs at this time.

3. Starvation, sepsis, and negative nitrogen balance are the critical factors if the patient survives the first two phases. A negative nitrogen balance exists because of the tissue injury (and subsequent tissue breakdown), loss of plasma in the exudate, severe loss of intracellular potassium, starvation, and continued stress. Nutritional sustenance, therefore, is a critical factor in the patient's survival. Whole blood transfusions are usually necessary to replace the body proteins lost with the plasma, thereby helping to reestablish a positive nitrogen balance. Potassium is usually administered intravenously, diluted in solution, to replace that which was lost. However, before potassium is given, it must be ascertained that the kidneys are functioning adequately.

4. Positive nitrogen balance. Nutrition becomes the key to recovery. A positive nitrogen balance will occur with sufficient nitrogen and caloric intake. Tube feedings may be necessary.

BLOOD ANALYSIS IN BURN SHOCK

Laboratory analysis of the patient's blood shows the following:

Increased hematocrit
Hemoconcentration (due to the concentration of hemoglobin)
Increased serum potassium

Azotemia (negative nitrogen balance)

Normal sodium chloride concentrations (which does not reflect
the total loss of body sodium—a patient may be dying because
of the lack of sodium, and yet the serum concentration may
be within normal limits)

SIGNS AND SYMPTOMS

The signs and symptoms exhibited by the patient in burn shock
are the direct result of the abnormal processes taking place within
the body—the losses of plasma, water, and electrolytes. Although these
signs and symptoms closely approximate those of the patient in hemorrhagic shock, there are a few exceptions which will be explained.

1. Inflammation of the affected area (heat, swelling, redness,
   loss of function).
2. Pain may or may not be present. Patients with third-degree
   burns usually do not have pain, because the nerve endings
   in the burned area are destroyed.
3. Anxiety and apprehension.
4. The state of consciousness may range from complete consciousness to semiconsciousness to unconsciousness.
5. The patient may feel faint.
6. Skin of unburned areas is pale, cool, and may be clammy.
   However, and this is important, because of a relative poly-
   cythemia, the patient's face may be flushed.
7. Complaints of thirst.
8. Nausea and vomiting are common.
9. Increasing pulse rate, thready or imperceptible.
10. Increasing respirations.
11. Increased body temperature.
12. Weakness.
13. Confusion.
14. Impaired capillary filling. Collapse or constriction of superfi-
    cial veins.
15. Oliguria or anuria.
16. Decreasing blood pressure.

An important point concerning the blood pressure of the patient
in burn shock must be made at this time. The blood pressure of patients
in shock due to a loss of plasma from the blood stream does not fall

185

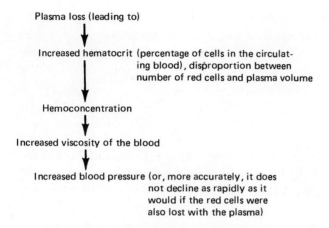

Plasma loss (leading to)

Increased hematocrit (percentage of cells in the circulating blood), disproportion between
number of red cells and plasma volume

Hemoconcentration

Increased viscosity of the blood

Increased blood pressure (or, more accurately, it does
not decline as rapidly as it
would if the red cells were
also lost with the plasma)

in proportion to the decrease of circulating fluid volume. (This also applies to other patients in shock due to a loss of plasma.) With the loss of plasma, the blood pressure remains higher than it would if the loss were whole blood. This is due to the increased blood viscosity which is explained in the above chain of events:

IMPLICATIONS FOR TREATMENT AND NURSING CARE

The critical period of shock usually lasts from 48 to 72 hours after the patient is burned. The immediate objectives and principles of nursing care for the patient in burn shock are the same as those for the patient in hemorrhagic shock:

1. Provide for the continuous flow of blood to the brain.
2. Facilitate respirations.
3. Provide for adequate blood volume and circulation of blood to all body tissues.
4. Provide for adequate nutrition of body cells.
5. Support and maintain the body's compensatory mechanisms, insofar as possible.
6. Relieve pain.

You will note that the objectives are arranged differently than those of the hemorrhaging patient. Priorities of patient-needs should dictate the sequence of objectives; when the priorities change, the objectives must be rearranged. The treatment and nursing care must fit the individual patient, and not necessarily follow the sequence as presented in this, or any other book.

Humidified oxygen and suctioning of the nasopharymx may be needed to ensure a clear airway. If the blood pressure is stable, cough and deep breathe the patient every 20 to 30 minutes. The patient should be turned at least every hour.

Blood gas determinations are indicated to assess treatment. If pulmonary damage is present, bronchodilators, antibiotics, and steroids may be indicated to decrease the inflammatory process.

INTAKE AND OUTPUT:

Intravenous fluids

While whole blood is the solution of choice for the hemorrhaging patient to achieve objective #3, plasma or a plasma expander and electrolytes are usually indicated for the patient in burn shock, since his hypovolemia is due mainly to a loss of plasma fluid and electrolytes. Later, as the integrity of the capillaries returns to normal, fluids and electrolytes remobilize into the vascular compartment from the interstitial compartment. Intravenous fluids are then changed accordingly, i.e., dextrose and water are usually given instead of plasma fluids and electrolytes. The patient should *never* be overloaded with fluids.

In recent years, hypertonic lactated saline (HLS) has become increasingly popular for the treatment of burned patients. Unlike Ringer's Lactate, hypertonic lactated saline reduces the average fluid load and weight gain from edema. Since the sodium concentration increases with the administration of HLS, the patient should be observed for cerebral symptoms.

Still another theory is that isotonic solutions reverse burn shock and minimize weight-gain. Such a solution is Ringer's Lactate with an addition of $NaHCO_3$. The use of normal saline for the treatment of the burned patient is contraindicated, as it contributes to the development of hyperchloremia and metabolic acidosis.

Oral fluids

Burn patients usually complain of thirst. Although some physicians may not wish the patient to have oral fluids, others may order a water and electrolyte solution to be given orally. Such a solution might be one-third sodium lactate (or citrate, or bicarbonate), and two-thirds sodium chloride mixed with water. If nausea and vomiting are present, it might be ordered to give this solution by intubation.

Tap water, which is a hypotonic solution, is contraindicated during the first 48 hours after the burn injury, as water intoxication, hence overhydration of the cells, can result. This is characterized by headache, loss of visual acuity, diarrhea, vomiting, oliguria, muscle twitching, apathy, and, in some severe cases, in seizures and death.

Output

Criteria used to determine the amount and type of intake (oral, intravenous, or intubation) the patient needs are usually the laboratory analysis of the patient's blood and the concentration and amount of his urine. The most satisfactory guides to determine the type and quantity of fluids needed are (1) the clinical condition of the patient, and (2) his urinary volume output. An adequate urinary output is considered to be between 30 and 50 ml. per hour. As soon as, but not until, a reasonable urinary output has been established, the patient's potassium should be replaced. Excretion of potassium is mainly through the kidneys. In the presence of oliguria, or anuria, potassium tends to accumulate in the extracellular fluid and may lead to potassium intoxication, which, in turn, could lead to cardiac arrest.

An accurate intake and output record must be made. Approximations are out of order; measurements down to the milliliter should be made. With the insertion of a Foley catheter, there is no reason why the output cannot be collected and measured accurately. The catheter can be connected to a tube emptying into a receptacle that is calibrated accurately in minims or milliliters. The same minute accuracy should be maintained in the measurement of the fluid intake. Along with hourly measurements of renal output, the specific gravity of the urine should also be measured. A low specific gravity (1.000 to 1.005) may indicate an overload of fluid; a high reading (1.020 to 1.030) may indicate that the patient needs more fluid.

Oliguria is usually present in the burn patient. The main reason for this is due to decreased cardiac output, hence decreased glomerular filtration rate. Secondarily, increased aldosterone and antidiuretic hormone contribute to this. An output of 30 ml. per hour indicates effective intravenous fluid resuscitation. In some instances, 600 to 700 ml. of intravenous fluid are necessary to maintain a urine output between 30 to 50 ml. per hour.

CRITERIA USED IN ADEQUACY OF TREATMENT

The adequacy of treatment of the patient in burn shock is attested by the following:

Stabilization of circulation
Correction of the hematocrit
Establishment of a satisfactory urinary output
Return of venous filling to the extremities
Return of warmth and color to the skin.

Potassium replacement

Because of extensive cellular destruction and damage, potassium diuresis may be excessive in shock due to burns and trauma, providing the kidneys are producing urine. This, of course, could lead to a marked hypokalemia (hypopotassemia). The serum potassium level may be lower than 4 mEq. per liter. The normal serum potassium averages 4 to 5 mEq per liter, (16 to 22 mg per 100cc of serum). Signs of hypokalemia are:

Muscle weakness (including the myocardium)
Dyspnea with gasping respirations
Anorexia
Nausea and vomiting
Distention
Chronic ileus
Cardiac failure.

It has been mentioned that potassium therapy usually is begun when the urinary output is satisfactory (30 to 50 ml. per hour). When potassium is administered intravenously, it should be given at a slow rate. Whether it is given intravenously or orally, the nurse must be alert to observe for possible signs and symptoms of hypokalemia or hyperkalemia. For parenteral use, potassium chloride (KCl) is supplied in ampules containing 30 or 40 mEq of potassium. One ampule is usually added to 1 liter of solution (electrolyte, glucose, or amino acid). It should be given slowly, so that the patient receives not more than 20 mEq per hour, or as indicated otherwise by the attending physician.

Potassium excess (hyperkalemia, potassium intoxication)

In the presence of oliguria, or anuria during the acute phase of shock, the body retains an excessive amount of potassium, and potassium intoxication may occur. It also can develop from an overdose of potassium. Signs of hyperkalemia are:

Cardiac irregularities of rate and rhythm
Peripheral vascular collapse
Cardiac arrest.

Treatment consists of immediate discontinuance of the drug and attempts to increase the urinary output. In the event that potassium intoxication occurs when the patient has acute renal failure, dialysis may be necessary.

ICE WATER AS AN EMERGENCY TREATMENT FOR BURNS

According to Mort, when a person is burned, regardless of the cause, "not all of the damage is done at once; the pathological process continues for at least three days."[10] The most valuable emergency first aid treatment is the immersion of the burned part into ice water. If the burns are on the face, neck, shoulders, or trunk, cold wet towels should be applied and changed frequently. Salt should *not* be added to the water, as frost bite could occur.

Occupational Health Nurses in the United States attest to the value of ice water treatment for burns, as they encounter many burned employees and have seen remarkable results.

Ice water slows down, or stops the pathological process, if used immediately following the burn. If the burn is due to chemicals, phisophex (or soap, if phisophex is not available) should be added to the water to flush the chemical from the skin. If possible, the area should be scrubbed.

Ice water treatment should be continued as long as the person has pain. Sometimes this may be as long as 12 to 24 hours.

ALTERATION OF THE PATHOLOGICAL PROCESS WITH THE USE OF ICE WATER

The application of ice water to burns:

1. Decreases pain.
2. Constricts the arteriolar blood vessels in the burned area, thus decreasing the capillary hydrostatic pressure and the amount of plasma fluid entering the interstitial compartment. The colloid osmotic pressure of the blood is maintained, and the incidence of interstitial edema is decreased.

---

[10] Eleanor H. Mort. "Cold Water Helps Healing of Burns," *Industrial Supervisor* (Dec. 1974), 10–12.

3. Decreases intracellular edema and the abnormal movement of electrolytes.
4. Decreases the incidence of infection.

SEVERE TRAUMA

Trauma is one of the most common causes of hypovolemic shock and, in many instances, is caused by frank hemorrhage. Traumatic shock, however, can occur without hemorrhage. Severe and/or extensive contusions to the body can cause sufficient damage to the capillaries, which, in turn, results in increased capillary permeability with a subsequent escape of plasma from the vascular compartment into the interstitial compartment. The implications are the same as those previously mentioned—decrease in circulating blood volume, disproportion between the hydrostatic pressure and the colloid osmotic pressure in the vascular compartment, and an abnormal increase of the colloid osmotic pressure within the interstitial compartment. Hence, there is a further reduction in blood volume and an increased blood viscosity.

Severe pain, often caused by trauma, can aggravate the degree of shock through its strong inhibitory effect on the vasomotor center which leads to an increased dilatation of peripheral vessels. Thus, a blood pressure that has already been decreased becomes even lower, and a further decrease in venous return occurs. Although traumatic shock results primarily from a decreased circulating blood volume, a concomitant neurogenic shock often accompanies and accentuates the shock condition.

The signs and symptoms of such a patient would closely resemble those of the patient in shock due solely to the loss of whole blood. However, there may be a few exceptions; for instance, the pulse might feel full, but weak, and the veins might be distended and would collapse when digital pressure is applied—due to the decreased volume of circulating blood and the massive vasodilatation. With a loss of circulating blood volume and the dysfunction of the important vasoconstrictive compensatory mechanisms the course of shock would be more rapid.

Two objectives of treatment are primary. (1) Provide for an adequate replacement of circulating blood volume. If the loss of fluid is chiefly plasma, plasma or a plasma expander is indicated. Vasoconstrictor drugs, in all probability, also will be administered in order to increase the arterial blood pressure and to increase the return of venous blood to the heart. (2) Provide for the relief of pain. When the patient is relieved of severe pain, his vasomotor center may be able to take over on its own, and the vasoconstrictor drugs may be discontinued. Another main objective is the provision of adequate respiratory exchange of gases. The reader is referred to the section dealing with hemorrhagic shock, where a thorough explanation was given.

Regardless of the cause, large losses of plasma result in:

Decreased blood volume.

A greatly increased blood viscosity which adds to the sluggishness of blood flow.

Certain characteristic metabolic and endocrine responses occur after traumatic injury. These are:

1. A negative nitrogen balance, due to the breakdown of body protein which is due to the injured tissues themselves, as well as to increased levels of endogenous corticosteriods. The corticosteroids cause gluconeogenesis by breaking down fats and proteins, and is followed by a loss of body weight. This negative nitrogen balance lasts from four to five days, depending on the severity of the injury. Initially, the nitrogen loss, which may amount to 12 to 15 gms. daily, cannot be replaced by an increased protein diet. When an increase in strength is exhibited by the patient, it is usually an indication that the nitrogen balance is returning to normal. Hyperalimentation fluids are often administered to rebuild the patient's nutritional status.

2. Loss of potassium (due to cell injury) creating a negative potassium balance for two or three days.

3. Low urinary excretion of sodium. This is due to the effects of increased aldosterone. Sodium, however, can be lost from the wound, or, if vomiting occurs, from the gastrointestinal tract.

4. Sympatho-adrenal medullary discharges are reflected clinically by tachycardia, vasoconstriction, and diaphoresis.

The traumatized area can be a portal of entry for pathogenic organisms.

Nonspecific effects of trauma can have a great influence on the following:

1. Central nervous system, resulting in depression, loss of consciousness, restlessness, hyperactivity, apprehension, delirium,

and convulsions. These could be due to hypoxia, infections, electrolyte disturbances, and/or renal impairment.

2. Liver in the form of impaired function. Hepatic insufficiency implies a decreased body resistance, decreased protein synthesis which leads to decreased fibrin and thrombin, which, in turn, leads to impaired coagulation of the blood.

IMPORTANT ASPECTS OF NURSING CARE AND TREATMENT

1. Assess level of consciousness.
2. An initial inspection of the patient should be made for evidence of severe injury requiring immediate attention.
3. Make sure the patient is breathing. Suction vomitus or blood that may be blocking the airway. Be sure the tongue is not obstructing the airway.
4. Look for chest wounds. Is there any evidence of mediastinal shift, pneumothorax, or paradoxical respirations.
5. Check for bleeding. If observed, apply direct pressure (if bleeding is from torso), or a tourniquet, if an extremity is involved. (Make sure you can feel an arterial pulse below the applied tourniquet.)
6. Keep patient in a supine position, unless contraindicated (such as in brain injury).
7. Do *not* overheat the patient.
8. Check vital signs and neuro signs (if indicated) every 10 to 15 minutes.
9. Insert urinary catheter and measure output hourly.

This list represents a different format than the other clinical examples presented in this book. From your understanding of physiology and altered physiology thus far, see if you can answer the following questions pertaining to the trauma patient.

1. What signs and symptoms of hypoxia might be present?
2. What are probable causes of hypoxia? (See Chapter 4.)
3. Explain the physiological implications of a pneumothorax. (Explanation of pneumothorax will be discussed later, but try it now anyway).
4. How would you know that the following are being produced? What parameters would you check in connection with this?

a. Norepinephrine
b. Epinephrine
c. Antidiuretic hormone
5. How much urine do the normal kidneys produce?
6. If the patient's BP is 90/40, what is his mean arterial pressure? (M.A.P.)
7. What are some signs of potassium deficiency?
8. Why is the trauma patient hyperglycemic?
9. What might lead you to suspect that the patient has an infection?
10. If whole blood is not available, what other solutions would be indicated? Why?

Diabetic Shock

Diabetic shock (coma, acidosis) is another example of hematogenic shock. It is characterized by metabolic acidosis and severe dehydration of all three fluid compartments—the vascular, interstitial, and intracellular.

Unlike the hemorrhagic shock patient, whose main treatment is the replacement of blood, and unlike the traumatic and burn shock patients, whose main treatment is the replacement of plasma fluid and electrolytes, the patient in diabetic shock requires something else in addition to the replacement of fluids and electrolytes—he requires insulin. Without insulin, his shock condition can only terminate in death.

In terms of the scope of this book, a thorough discussion of diabetes mellitus would be out of order. However, in order to understand the physiologic mechanisms involved in diabetic shock and in the period immediately preceding it, a certain background of information is essential.

DIABETES MELLITUS

Diabetes mellitus is a metabolic disorder characterized by a lack of insulin in the body which, in turn, causes an inability of the body cells to utilize glucose for energy, and an inability of the liver and muscle cells to store glucose as glycogen. The onset of diabetes mellitus is gradual in adults and acute in children. Early signs and symptoms are:

Loss of weight
Loss of strength
Polyuria (excessive urination)
Polydipsia (excessive thirst)
Polyphagia (excessive hunger)
Itchy, dry skin

PRINCIPLE 44:   All body cells require energy for their activity.
PRINCIPLE 45:   Human energy is derived from the oxidation of foods.

Foods + $O_2 \rightarrow CO_2 + H_2O$ + energy (heat)
(carbon compounds:
carbohydrates
fats
proteins).

Carbohydrate in the form of glucose is the most readily available source
of energy in the body.

GLUCOSE

Glucose is the main source from which energy is derived, and,
in nondiabetic individuals, it is freely utilized in the process of cellular
metabolism. If the amount of glucose in our bodies is more than we
need at any one time, the excess is stored mainly in the liver and
also in the muscle cells as glycogen. Some glucose also might be converted into fat and stored for future use as fuel. Thereafter, if our
intake of foods is low, our liver, muscle cells, and fat stores release
glucose into the blood stream to be used in producing energy.

CARBOHYDRATES, FATS, AND PROTEINS

Although energy can be derived from carbohydrates, fats, and
proteins, it is not usually necessary for the body to use protein as a
source of energy.

Carbohydrates taken into the body are converted into glucose.
Fat is broken down by the digestive juices into fatty acids and glycerol,
before it is absorbed into the system. The glycerol component of the
fat molecule can be converted into glucose. In the normal combustion
of fats and carbohydrates, carbon dioxide, water, and energy are liber-
ated. In the process of fat oxidation, fatty byproducts of acetoacetic

195

acid and beta-hydroxybutyric acid are produced. Normally, the oxidation of these two acids is complete; however, in uncontrolled diabetes mellitus they cannot be entirely oxidized to carbon dioxide and water. Therefore, the accumulation of these two acids in the body leads to an acid intoxication which causes much of the damage occurring in this disease.

Protein, of which nitrogen is the chief characteristic element, is normally concerned with the structural integrity and life of the cell. When digested into the body, protein splits up into many different kinds of amino acids. Although the chief function of protein is to build and repair body tissues, some of its amino acids are capable of being broken down to glucose and burned to yield energy. If the protein is used to provide energy, however, it cannot perform its own unique function. As a result, the structural integrity of body tissue cells suffers to the extent of cell injury with subsequent tissue breakdown. An increased rate of protein catabolism leads to a negative nitrogen balance, delayed healing, and increased susceptibility to infections.

THE ROLE OF INSULIN IN THE BODY

PRINCIPLE 46: The utilization of fuel is necessary for the proper functioning of body cells.

It is a cold, wintry day. Your cabin is isolated in the north woods. In order to heat the cabin, you must build a fire in the fireplace. You place the fuel in the grate, but before it can burn and yield heat (energy), it must be ignited. So you strike a match to the fuel, and soon you have a nice glowing fire which provides warmth for you. Without the match to ignite the fuel, however, you would not have a fire.

Insulin can be compared to the match in the above analogy. Without insulin, our glucose (fuel) could not be oxidized by our body cells to yield energy. Also, without insulin, extra supplies of glucose could not be stored for future use.

Now let us suppose that you laid the materials for the fire and discovered that you had no match with which to ignite it. Consequently (but not very wisely, I might add), you break up the furniture and pile it in the fireplace. You discover, however, that without a match to ignite it, your efforts are useless. Somewhat desperately, you start to tear down the cabin to use the wood for fuel—with the same fruitless results. Unless you can find a match, the inevitable will occur—you will freeze to death.

* The severely diabetic individual, in comparison with the above analogy, will draw on his stores of carbohydrate, fat, and protein, but without insulin he will be unable to generate heat and energy at the cellular level; hence, his efforts will be in vain. Unless insulin is administered to the patient in diabetic shock (acidosis), this destructive process cannot be reversed, and death will be inevitable.

ᛁ Insulin in the body, therefore, serves two purposes: (1) its presence in the blood stream is required for the oxidation of foods to take place in the cells, and (2) its presence is required for the storage of extra glucose supplies in the liver and muscle cells.

What, then, happens to the glucose if it cannot be used by the cells, and if it cannot be stored in the liver and muscle cells? Decreased production of insulin causes a decreased metabolism of glucose in most body tissues. Since the glucose from carbohydrates available in the body cannot be utilized for energy, it accumulates in the blood stream and is spilled out into the urine. Blood and urine tests show hyperglycemia and glycosuria, respectively.

ABNORMAL METABOLISM OF FATS

When the glucose stores of the liver and muscle cells have been depleted (analogous to the fuel in the fireplace), there is a shift from carbohydrate to fat metabolism (analogous to the broken-up furniture). The fats are broken down to glycerol and fatty acids. From the glycerol, glucose is made available, but (again) in the absence of insulin in the blood stream, the glucose cannot reach the cells to provide energy. The fatty acids—acetoacetic acid and beta-hydroxybutyric acid—are not oxidized properly, and they accumulate in the blood stream in large quantities, causing metabolic acidosis and sodium diuresis. Therefore, with the loss of large amounts of sodium bicarbonate from the extracellular fluids, large amounts of fluid accompany it and are excreted in the urine. A small amount of acetoacetic acid can be converted to acetone, which is volatile and is vaporized into the air on the expiratory phase of breathing. This accounts for the fruity-sweet odor of the breath of the patient in diabetic acidosis.

With the progression into metabolic acidosis, which is characterized by incomplete metabolism of fats, one of the major effects is depression of the central nervous system. (Before acidosis sets in, however, the individual is usually conscious and alert, because brain cells do not require insulin for the normal utilization of glucose.) When the pH of the blood falls below 7.0, the nervous system becomes so depressed that disorientation and coma develop.

In health, the hydrogen ion concentration in the blood is maintained within the pH range of 7.35 to 7.45 units. A pH value of less than 7.35 represents acidosis, while a pH above 7.45 represents alkalosis. If the pH of body fluids falls below approximately 7.0 to 6.9, the diabetic may develop coma.

ABNORMAL PROTEIN METABOLISM

Since the body cannot derive energy from its carbohydrates and fats, it begins to tear down its own structure (analogous to tearing down the cabin), in an effort to use protein as fuel. Although many of the protein amino acids can be converted into glucose to be used for energy, unless the body is supplied with sufficient insulin, it will not be able to utilize any of the glucose from the protein, either. In a word, the body's efforts are commendable, but fruitless.

EFFECTS OF HYPERGLYCEMIA

The only significant effect of a very high blood-glucose level is dehydration of the tissues and cells, i.e., dehydration of the interstitial and intracellular compartments. The increased crystalloidal osmotic pressure effect exerted in the vascular compartment is the direct result of the increased amount of glucose in the blood stream. Therefore, fluids from the interstitial and intracellular compartments are drawn into the blood stream and excreted by the kidneys.* This, coupled with the loss of body sodium, means that large quantities of body fluids are lost (with an obligatory loss of electrolytes), which leaves the body in a state of marked dehydration.

A PATIENT IN DIABETIC SHOCK

Mrs. Doris Matthews, sixty-three years of age, was admitted to the hospital in diabetic acidosis and coma. She was accompanied by her son, who found her in bed at home where she lives alone.

* The normal renal threshold for glucose is about 160 mg. When the blood sugar rises above this level, the excess overflows into the urine. The presence of sugar in the urine is called glycosuria. Hyperglycemia and glycosuria are two of the cardinal signs of diabetes mellitus.

According to Mr. Matthews, his mother has been a known diabetic for nine years, and, to his knowledge, she had never been in diabetic coma before. He had talked with his mother on the telephone three days ago, and she had mentioned that she had a cold. Other than that and a sore toe, she had no complaints.

Mr. Matthews told the doctor: "When I rang the door bell, mother didn't answer like she usually does, so, thinking she might be at the store, I let myself into the house with the key she had given me. When I stepped into the house, I smelled a fruity-sweet odor; it smelled much like fingernail-polish remover. I thought this rather odd, because mother never uses fingernail polish. Then I heard a noise coming from the bedroom. I dashed in there and discovered mother lying in bed. She looked thinner than she looked last week, and her skin was wrinkled and dry. She acted as though she was drugged, or inebriated. She tried to focus her eyes on me as she muttered almost inaudibly, 'I'm thirsty.' I brought her a glass of water and, as I helped her to sit up in bed, I noticed that she was very weak. She seemed to know me, as she said my name and told me how dizzy she felt. Then she became drowsy, and I put her back down in bed. I was afraid she was dead, but then I noticed that she was breathing very deeply, yet not with any difficulty. I phoned for our family doctor, but he was out on a house-call, so I phoned for an ambulance, and it arrived in ten minutes. When we lifted mother out of bed onto the stretcher, I saw that she had urinated a lot in bed, but the bed linen was pretty well dried with the urine stain. At any rate, I don't think she had urinated within the past few hours. What do you think is wrong with her, doctor?" To which the doctor replied, "She's in diabetic shock." "But," said Mr. Matthews, "I just saw her three days ago, and she was all right then." The doctor replied, "But that was 72 hours ago. I would judge this condition started approximately 24 to 36 hours ago, until it has progressed to this severe stage."

From this history, the doctor made the diagnosis of shock due to diabetic acidosis and coma. He began treatment immediately. Although he did not wait for the laboratory report on the blood studies before he started treatment, these studies showed the following:

Hyperglycemia
Low CO_2-combining power
Increased keto acids, increased acidity
Increased cholesterol

Elevated NPN
Decreased chlorides
Decreased sodium
Decreased potassium.

Urine obtained from a catheter showed:

4-plus sugar
Positive acetone.

The signs and symptoms reported by Mr. Matthews were:

Acetone odor to breath
Emaciation
Dry skin
Thirst
Drowsiness and listlessness
Visual disturbances, difficulty in focusing
Dizziness
Weakness
Kussmaul's respirations
Polyuria, followed by oliguria
Finally, unconsciousness.

Besides these signs and symptoms, the following might also occur:

Nausea and/or vomiting
Anorexia
Headache
Abdominal pain and gastric dilatation
Tinnitus
Excitement or delirium.

IMPLICATIONS FOR TREATMENT AND NURSING CARE

The main medical objective in treating the patient in diabetic shock resulting from metabolic acidosis is to restore an insulin-glucose-water-electrolyte balance. With this underway, the metabolic deficiencies resulting from insulin insufficiency—dehydration and decreased cellular utilization of glucose for energy—will be corrected.

The decreased blood pressure of the patient is the result of a decreased blood volume caused by the severe dehydration of the body, which, in turn, resulted from the diuretic effects of hyperglycemia and sodium loss. Insulin deficiency, of course, is the primary factor responsible for this chain of events. The recovery of the patient is dependent on the coordinated vigilance and purposeful actions of the nursing and medical staffs.

OBJECTIVES AND PRINCIPLES OF NURSING CARE

Most often, the nurse's and doctor's first encounter with the patient in diabetic shock is on the patient's admission to the hospital. In such instances, the doctor should be accompanied by a nurse, as there is much she can do while he is getting a quick history from a relative or friend of the patient. At such a time, the nurse should anticipate the immediate needs of the patient and take the necessary steps toward alleviating them. The nurse who sees nothing to do for the patient, while she waits for the doctor's orders, is the nurse who has a poor understanding of diabetic shock. For example, while the doctor is getting the history, the nurse can check for any signs of respiratory obstruction and take the necessary steps to remove it through oronasal suctioning. Also, she should see that the patient is lying flat. She can check the vital signs. If she is not new to diabetic nursing, she probably will recognize the sweet acetone odor of the patient's breath. This recognition, along with the history, can well furnish the main clue for the diagnosis and subsequent treatment.

OBJECTIVE 1: Maintain a patent airway.
PRINCIPLE 47: Among other things, adequate exchange of respiratory gases is dependent on a clear airway.

Suctioning of the nasal passages, pharynx, and larynx should be done immediately in the presence of wet or noisy breathing. The appropriate equipment should be readily accessible for immediate use.

OBJECTIVE 2: Provide for increased circulation of blood to the brain.
Lay victim flat
Even though the abnormal constituents within the patient's blood stream will not contribute to adequate nutrition of the brain cells, the oxygen in the blood is needed most vitally by the brain tissues. For this reason, the patient's position should be flat, in order to decrease the resistance to the flow of blood to the brain.

OBJECTIVE 3: Provide for the physiologic replacement and balance of insulin, glucose, hydration, and electrolytes to body tissues.

201

a. Provide for adequate metabolism of glucose.

b. Provide for adequate fluid and electrolyte balance.

PRINCIPLE 48: The life and proper functioning of all body tissues are dependent on adequate nutrition.

PRINCIPLE 49: The metabolism of glucose in the human body (with the exception of brain tissue) is dependent on a sufficient amount of insulin in the blood stream.

PRINCIPLE 50: A proportional balance of fluids and electrolytes within the body is basic to health.

• Usually, before insulin and fluid therapies are begun, a urine specimen is obtained (unless the patient is anuric). Since this patient is in coma, the insertion of a catheter will be necessary and should be left in place. •As soon as a fresh sample of urine is obtained, it should be tested for sugar and acetone. A blood test usually is taken by the physician at the time he starts parenteral treatment, and it is sent to the laboratory to be tested primarily for sugar and electrolytes. •On the basis of history and the initial urine test, treatment is started. The main medical objective is to correct the hyperglycemia, dehydration, and electrolyte imbalance. These will be corrected by the administration of insulin and intravenous solutions of glucose and electrolytes.

Ideally, although each dose of insulin should depend on a blood sugar determination, this is rarely practicable. Unless anuria exists, generally it is considered quite satisfactory to regulate the amount of insulin to be given on the basis of hourly urine examinations for glycosuria and acetone. To protect the patient from hypoglycemia, which could prove fatal, sufficient glucose often is administered in the intraveous solution. Only a quick-acting insulin should be given to patients in diabetic acidosis, and it should be given deep intramuscularly with an intramuscular needle. It is advocated that if the patient is in profound shock, the insulin should be injected directly into a vein and not put into the infusion solution. In severe cases, insulin may be ordered to be given every half hour, in less severe cases, at one- or two-hour intervals. Half-hourly injections usually are ordered to be continued until the acetone in the urine declines to 1 or 2+, and the patient shows signs of clinical improvement.

This is one example of insulin replacement, but it is by no means the *only* method of management. The main point to remember, however, is that the orders should be followed explicitly and on time.

Since considerable amounts of sodium, chlorides, and potassium have been lost, fluids containing these electrolytes are administered intravenously, as a rule. It is well to repeat, however, that potassium is withheld until the urine output is satisfactory. Also, if potassium is given too rapidly, hyperkalemia and cardiac arrest might occur.

Whole blood or plasma transfusions may be necessary to repair cellular loss, especially in the case of the severely dehydrated patient who has been in ketosis for more than 12 hours.

At any rate, the nursing care involved for the achievement of Objective 3 is:

Retention catheter is inserted.

Urine is tested for sugar and acetone, and results are recorded and reported.

The insulin and intravenous solutions ordered are prepared, and the electrolytes ordered are added to the solution.

The insulin is administered.

Assistance is given for the administration of parenteral fluids.

The patient's extremity is secured to prevent the needle from slipping out of the vein.

The quantity of urinary output is checked; a thorough and accurate record of the intake and output is kept.

When the body once again is able to utilize its glucose for energy and to store excess glucose in the liver and muscle cells, the abnormal metabolism of fat is arrested, and the fatty acids in the blood stream begin to disappear. At this time, the acetone content in the urine will also decline. The abnormal metabolism of protein stops, and, once again, the protein can be utilized for the growth and repair of body tissues.

OBJECTIVE 4:   Provide for an adequate blood volume and blood pressure.

PRINCIPLE 51:   The proper functioning of all body tissues is dependent on a sufficient volume of blood flowing under sufficient pressure.

Mrs. Matthews' decreased blood pressure is caused by a decreased blood volume, which in turn is caused by a state of marked dehydration resulting from hyperglycemia and sodium and water diuresis. With the administration of parenteral fluids and electrolytes (mentioned in Objective 3) her blood volume will increase, and there will be a subsequent elevation of her blood pressure. The blood pressure and pulse should be checked and recorded at least every 15 minutes.

OBJECTIVE 5:   Provide for intelligent observation of the patient.

A nurse should be in constant attendance of the patient in diabetic shock (coma). Coma is not an independent disease, but rather it is a symptom of disease. Coma varies in degree, and in its deepest stage there is no reaction of any kind from the patient. The patient in coma appears to be asleep; however, he is incapable of sensing or responding to external stimuli. The cause of diabetic coma is a decreased pH of the blood, resulting from acidosis. This, in turn, exerts a marked depressant effect on the central nervous system.

The patient with marked dehydration will have dry skin, tongue, and mucous membranes. As soon as time permits, the nurse should give special mouth care to the patient. This, however, should not take precedence over the more vital, specific needs of the patient.

Soft eyeballs, due to reduced intraocular tension, are also often present in the severely dehydrated patient. In coma, the patient's eyes will tend to diverge slightly. In light coma, the patient's eyes often can be induced to move to either side by turning his head. If the head is turned to the right, the eyes will move to the left. If the head is turned to the left, the eyes will move to the right. These simple tests can be done by the nurse to determine the degree of coma. Once treatment is instituted (insulin, glucose, and electrolyte solution) the nurse should be observant for any sign that the patient is coming out of the comatose state.

In a comatose state, the patient is totally unable to tend to any of his own needs; this must be done for him by the nurse. The patient's respirations should be checked carefully. Suctioning should be done as necessary. The nature of the respirations should be noted. Kussmaul's respirations are indicative of diabetic acidosis and are characterized by deep, rapid, unlabored breathing. Kussmaul's respirations also appear in patients who are suffering from uremic acidosis.

The nurse should understand the significance of different breathing patterns. For example, abnormally slow breathing is indicative of either morphine or barbiturate intoxication. Rapid breathing accompanied by an expiratory grunt and associated with fever is frequently found in patients with lobar pneumonia. Slow, irregular, or periodic breathing, referred to as Cheyne-Stokes respirations, is found in patients having diseases that cause an elevated intracranial pressure or damaged brain.

As the treatment takes effect, the patient will show signs of coming out of the coma. Before complete consciousness occurs, the patient may appear stuporous. Stupor is a state of reduced, but not necessarily absent, mental and physical activity. The patient can open his eyes, and at times he can respond slowly to spoken commands. At any rate, the nurse must be observant for the effectiveness of the treatment.

Mrs. Matthews' respiratory infection and her sore toe may have precipitated her state of diabetic shock. Antibiotics generally are prescribed to combat such infections.

If the patient's blood pressure does not rise, it may be necessary for the doctor to order a vasoconstrictor, such as norepinephrine. Special precautions should be taken while the patient is receiving such a drug.

The injections of insulin should be given in varied sites. If injections are given in the same area, lipodystrophy might occur. Lipodystrophy is characterized by a complete atrophy of the subcutaneous fat at the site of insulin injections. Localized deep hollows are produced in the skin. Such areas could decrease the absorption time of the insulin, besides predisposing to inflammatory reactions. Lipodystrophy is more prevalent in women and children than it is in men.

The nurse's role in caring for the patient in diabetic shock is not an easy one. Many procedures must be done in a short span of time. It is best to have all the equipment needed within easy access. If any equipment, solution, or insulin is needed that is not in the patient's room, the nurse should signal for assistance rather than leave the patient unattended. If she must leave the room, she should make certain that the patient is protected with side rails so that he cannot fall out of bed.

REFERENCES

Artz, Curtis P., Paulette Miller, and Elizabeth W. Bayley. "The Burned Patient: Current Concepts of Medical and Nursing Management" in *Advanced Concepts in Clinical Nursing* (Kay Corman Kintzel, ed.), Philadelphia: J. B. Lippincott, 1977, pp. 252–291.

Chaffee, Ellen, and Esther Greisheimer. *Basic Physiology and Anatomy*, 3rd Ed., Philadelphia: J. B. Lippincott, 1974.

Guyton, Arthur C. *Textbook of Medical Physiology*, 5th Ed., Philadelphia: W. B. Saunders, 1976.

Jarvis, Carolyn Mueller. "Vital Signs," *Nursing '76* (April 1976), 31–37.

Jones, C. A., and I. Feller. "Burns," *Nursing '77*, 7 (1977).

Jung, Omero and Franklin Wade. "The Treatment of Burns with Ice Water, Phisohex, and Partial Hypothermia," *Industrial Medicine and Surgery* (Sept. 1963), 365–370.

Langley, L. L. *Review of Physiology*, 3rd ed., New York: McGraw-Hill Book Co., 1971.

Lucas, Charles E. "Resuscitation of the Injured Patient: The Three Phases of Treatment," *Surgical Clinics of North America*, 57 (Feb. 1977), 3–15.

McCredie, John A. (ed.). *Basic Surgery*, New York: Macmillan Publishing Co., Inc., 1977.

Nadrowski, Leon F. "Pathophysiology and Current Treatment of Intestinal Obstruction," *Review of Surgery*, 31 (Nov.–Dec. 1974), 381.

Roach, Lora B. "Color Changes in Dark Skin," *Nursing '77*, 7 (Jan. 1977), 48–51.

Rogenes, P. R. and J. A. Moyland. "Restoring Fluid Balance in the Patient with Severe Burns," *American Journal of Nursing*, 76 (Dec. 1976), 1052–1057.

Rush, Jr., Benjamin F. "Volume Replacement: When, What, and How Much?," in *Treatment of Shock: Principles and Practice* (W. Schumer and Nyhus, eds.), Philadelphia: Lea and Febiger, 1974, pp. 23–36.

Secor, Jane. *Patient Care in Respiratory Problems*, Saunders Monograph in Clinical Nursing, Philadelphia: W. B. Saunders Co., 1969.

Shires, G. Tom (ed.). *Care of the Trauma Patient*, New York: McGraw-Hill Book Co., 1966.

Sodeman, William and William Sodeman, Jr., *Pathologic Physiology*, 5th ed., Philadelphia: W. B. Saunders Co., 1974.

Shulman, Alexander G. "Ice Water as Primary Treatment of Burns," *Journal of the American Medical Association*, 173 (Aug. 27, 1960), pp. 1916–1919.

Thal, Alan P., et al. *Shock*, Chicago: Year Book Medical Publishers, 1971.

CHAPTER 10

Cardiogenic Shock

Shock caused by heart failure is called *cardiogenic,* or *cardiac* shock. Heart failure represents the inability of the heart to pump blood in sufficient quantity to all parts of the body. The effects are the same as for hypovolemic shock, i.e., a decreased supply of oxygen, nutrients, water, electrolytes, and hormones to all body cells, and a decreased removal of waste products from the cells.

Causes of Cardiogenic Shock

Cardiogenic shock can result from any condition that leads to decreased cardiac output. Left myocardial infarction is the most common cause of cardiogenic shock. Less common causes are

Rupture of the interventricular septum
Rupture of a chorda papilla
Rupture of the ventricular wall with acute tamponade
Coronary embolus

Rupture of aortic aneurysm
Dissecting aortic aneurysm
Direct trauma to the heart
Serious cardiac arrhythmias
Shock related to cardiac surgery
Obstruction of venous inflow to the right atrium, such as occurs
    with:
  Tension pneumothorax
  Mediastinal shift
  Embolus in the vena cava
  Cardiac tamponade

In short, anything that decreases left ventricular output will cause cardiogenic shock.

Typical features of cardiogenic shock are the following:

1. Systolic blood pressure less than 90 mm. Hg. pressure (80 mm. Hg. per intra-arterial measurement).
2. Decreased blood flow, inclusive of decreased urinary output of less than 20 ml./hour, with a low sodium content.
3. Impaired mental function.
4. Peripheral vasoconstriction associated with cold, clammy skin.

The physiological ramifications of left myocardial failure are numerous. They will be discussed in detail in the following pages.

SIGNS OF HEART FAILURE: (LEFT-SIDED FAILURE)[1]

*Early signs**

Tachycardia
Gallop rhythm
Pulsus alternans
Left ventricular hypertrophy
Dyspnea
Orthopnea
Paroxysmal nocturnal dyspnea
Rales (fine, crepitant)
Cough
Fatigue, weakness, restlessness

[1] Tanner, Gloria. "Heart Failure in the M.I. Patient," *American Journal of Nursing* (Feb. 1977), 230–234.
* Note: A person in early or late heart failure does not necessarily exhibit *all* of these signs.

*Late signs**

Increasing fatigue, weakness, restlessness

Distended neck veins

Hepatojugular reflux

Oliguria

Anorexia, nausea, vomiting

Decreased blood pressure

Cheyne-Stokes respirations

Pulmonary edema

Hepatomegaly

If the basic physiology as presented in this text, is understood, the reader should be able to explain each of these signs, scientifically.

Cardiogenic Shock Due to Left Myocardial Failure

Mr. Henry John was admitted to the hospital in shock due to severe left myocardial failure. Let us trace the events of the day he was admitted to the hospital.

Mr. Henry John, fifty-seven years of age, is a salesman whose job entails considerable statewide travel. Mr. John is 5 ft 10 inches tall, and weighs 195 lb. Although he knows he is overweight, he does not curb his appetite for rich desserts, cream, butter, fatty meats, and other foods high in calories and cholesterol.

Much of the time he spends on his job consists of travel by train, plane, or bus; it seems as though he is in a continuous rush to meet time schedules. Often he gets overtired, not getting to sleep some nights until one or two o'clock in the morning. But he is well compensated for his job, despite the many annoyances that seem to accompany it.

Although the demands of Mr. John's position do not include heavy physical work, nevertheless, he is exposed to many stressful situations—the constant rush of travel, his mounting overweight, his efforts to please unreasonable clients, and, within the past few years, a nervous dissatisfied temperament which often is manifested in outbursts of anger at his family.

On the day of his heart attack, the following events occurred.

The month was December; the weather was cold. Mr. John was waiting for a bus. Because he had forgotten his gloves, his hands were in his pockets. He felt chilly. The bus was late. He glanced at his

* See footnote on p. 208.

watch. He wished the bus would come. He'd be late for an important business engagement. He waited. His exasperation increased. He could think of no alternative; at this time of year taxis were unavailable.

Traffic was heavy. A truck passed, and, as it made a sharp turn around a corner, a large box dropped off. The driver stopped as Mr. John yelled to him. Seeing no bus in sight, Mr. John ran to the corner, lifted the big, heavy box, and helped the driver put it back on the truck. He went back to his position at the bus stop.

Finally, he saw a bus coming. But because it was overcrowded, it did not stop. Mr. John became outraged. He vented his feelings to others around him. It was at this time that he had a severe heart attack. With a sudden shriek, he clutched his chest, and with a frightened wild-eyed stare he collapsed to the sidewalk in a state of unconsciousness. His face was very pale. He was brought to the hospital by a passing motorist, who loosened his collar and, with the help of another man, laid him flat on the back seat of the car.

By the time he reached the hospital, Mr. John was semiconscious and complained of severe shortness of breath and excruciating chest pain. His skin was cold, clammy, and pale. His lips and nail beds were cyanotic. He was confused and weak. His pulse was irregular and very weak. His arterial blood pressure was 90/70 mm. Hg. A diagnosis of cardiogenic shock due to left heart failure was made. It was subsequently determined that he had a left myocardial infarction due to a coronary artery occlusion.

Normal Versus Abnormal Left Heart Action

Keep the following facts in mind: Mr. John's left heart failed because of an occlusion of a left coronary artery, which prevented an adequate supply of blood from reaching a large part of his left myocardium. When it is deprived of an adequate blood supply (hence, receives decreased oxygen and nutrients), the ability of the left myocardium to contract is greatly diminished. Let us compare the normal actions of the left side of the heart to the physiologic implications of the abnormal actions.

NORMAL LEFT HEART ACTION

1. During systole:
    a. The left ventricle contracts and pumps oxygenated blood

into the aorta. From the aorta the blood is forced into other arteries, including the coronary arteries, and delivered to all parts of the body.

2. During diastole:
   a. Oxygenated blood from the lungs flows into the left atrium via the four pulmonary veins.
   b. Oxygenated blood flows from the left atrium into the left ventricle.
   c. Oxygenated blood in the coronary arteries flows into the right and left sides of the myocardium.

ABNORMAL LEFT HEART ACTION DUE TO MYOCARDIAL INSUFFICIENCY

1. During systole:
   a. A decreased quantity of poorly oxygenated blood is pumped by the left ventricle into the aorta, coronary arteries, and systemic arteries. (The degree to which the quantity of blood is decreased is relative to the strength of the left myocardium, which, in turn, is determined by the degree of coronary insufficiency.)
   b. Because of the weakened left myocardium, the left ventricle fails to empty completely.
2. During diastole:
   a. A very small quantity of poorly oxygenated blood enters the left myocardium from the left coronary artery because—
      (1) Coronary obstruction prevents the normal quantitative passage of blood into the myocardium, and
      (2) The quantity of blood ejected from the left ventricle into the aorta and coronary artery vessels is insufficient. Coronary blood flow is directly proportional to the diastolic blood pressure. If the diastolic blood pressure decreases to critical levels for a prolonged length of time, myocardial injury occurs and the patient may develop congestive heart failure or an arrhythmia; either of which may be fatal.
   b. Owing to the failure of the left ventricle to empty completely during systole, some blood remains in the left ventricular chamber, which causes—
      (1) A dilatation of the left ventricle, and
      (2) A damming up of blood up to the left atrium and the pulmonary venous circuit. As a consequence:

(a) The left atrium is dilated

(b) A decreased amount of oxygenated blood is delivered to the left atrium via the four pulmonary veins, and

(c) Pressure is increased within the pulmonary capillary bed, forcing plasma or whole blood into the pulmonary interstitial compartment and, finally, into the pulmonary alveoli.

With the perfusion of plasma, and sometimes red blood cells, across the pulmonary alveolar membranes, respiratory insufficiency ensues. Many of the alveoli, now either partially or totally filled with fluid, cannot carry on their normal function of diffusing oxygen and carbon dioxide. Thus, the pulmonary capillary blood stream is poorly oxygenated and overloaded with carbon dioxide. Blood that then flows to the left atrium and ventricle is a mixture of venous and arterial blood, and a state of hypercapnia and acidosis develops. The main systemic implication is a decreased quantity and quality of oxygenated blood to body tissues, resulting in tissue hypoxia. More imminently dangerous, of course, are the pulmonary effects of alveolar perfusion.

To add insult to injury, an insufficient quantity of oxygenated blood is delivered to the right myocardium, and, of course, to the left myocardium whose coronary artery is partially occluded. Consequently, the left myocardium, especially, becomes weaker and weaker,

Figure 22. *Pulmonary congestion due to left heart failure.*
A. Inspiration. Due to the perfusion of plasma into the alveolus, the surface area for the diffusion of gases is decreased; hence, less oxygen and carbon dioxide cross the membrane.
B. Expiration. Recoil of the alveolus is less than normal, due to the abnormal fluid content within the alveolus.

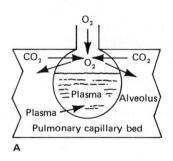
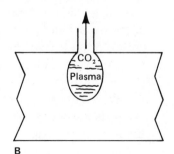

A

B

until a vicious cycle of cardiac deterioration progresses into cardiogenic shock. Unless adequate nursing care and medical treatment are instituted rapidly, death of the patient will ensue. And death often wins out, despite prompt nursing and medical attention. Pulmonary edema can develop so rapidly that it results in death only 10 to 20 minutes after the onset of the attack. Left heart failure, without right heart failure, leads to rapid pulmonary vascular congestion.

Pathologic Physiology

An obstruction to the flow of blood to any part of the body results in a decreased supply of blood, and hence a decreased supply of oxygen and nutrients to that particular area. Therefore, the deprived area becomes ischemic and is unable to perform normally. In the case of the left myocardium, which is responsible for pumping blood from the left heart chambers, weakness will occur in that part of the left myocardium deprived of a normal supply of blood. The following series of events occurs after a left myocardial infarction:

Obstruction of left coronary artery
Left myocardial insufficiency
Decreased strength of contraction of left myocardium
Decreased systolic emptying of left ventricle (increased LVEDP)
Increased residual blood in left ventricle
Dilatation of left ventricle
Damming up of blood in left atrium
Increased left atrial pressure and dilatation
Damming up of blood in the pulmonary veins
Pulmonary engorgement
Pulmonary edema
Perfusion of pulmonary alveoli with plasma fluid
Decreased diffusion of oxygen and carbon dioxide across alveolar
    membranes
Respiratory insufficiency
Severe dyspnea

The following sequence of events resulting from left heart failure shows its effects on the right side of the heart and the systemic circulation:

213

Left myocardial failure
Decreased cardiac output
Increased pressure in left atrium and ventricle
Decreased inflow of blood into left atrium from pulmonary veins
Increased accumulation of blood and pressure in pulmonary circuit
Damming up of blood in right side of heart
Incomplete emptying of blood into pulmonary artery from right ventricle
Increased pressure in right ventricle
Increased pressure in right atrium →* ↑CVP
Decreased inflow of blood from systemic veins (venae cavae) into right atrium
Elevation of venous pressure in systemic circuit.

There is, therefore, an accumulation of blood in the right heart chambers and in the great veins causing congestion. Subsequently, the circulating oxygenated blood in the peripheral vessels is deficient.

The incomplete emptying of the right side of the heart does not occur immediately after the failure of the left myocardium. Although left myocardial failure is characterized by an immediate failure of the left atrium and ventricle to empty completely, it should be emphasized that the nonaffected right side of the heart functions almost normally in the early period of the heart attack. Thus, from the right ventricle, blood is forced in normal amounts through the pulmonary artery to the lungs. This normal right heart action accounts for the increasing pressure in the pulmonary vascular bed, since the blood from the left heart chamber is dammed up to the pulmonary venous circuit. Later, when the right myocardium has become sufficiently weakened because of a poor supply of oxygenated blood from the right coronary artery, there is an accumulation of blood in the right heart chambers with a damming up of blood into the great veins.

In heart failure accompanied by peripheral failure (massive dilatation of peripheral blood vessels), the venous inflow load into the right atrium is decreased. In practically all other instances of heart failure, the venous inflow load is elevated. In all types of heart failure there is a decline in cardiac output relative to the inflow load of venous blood. It should be reemphasized that while absolute decline in cardiac

---

* → means "leads to."

output is not present in all cases, decline in cardiac output, relative to the venous inflow load does occur in all instances.

Compensatory Mechanisms; A Paradox

With the occurrence of heart failure, certain adjustments are made to compensate for the decreased cardiac output. While these adjustments are compensatory in one sense, in that they alleviate the decline in cardiac output, they are also harmful because they tend to aggravate the congestion (cardiopulmonary). Thus, the compensatory mechanisms involved tend to be more of a hindrance than a help in acute heart failure. Figure 23 is a schematic representation of this paradox.

Figure 23. *A schematic representation of the effects of compensatory mechanisms in heart failure—a paradox.*

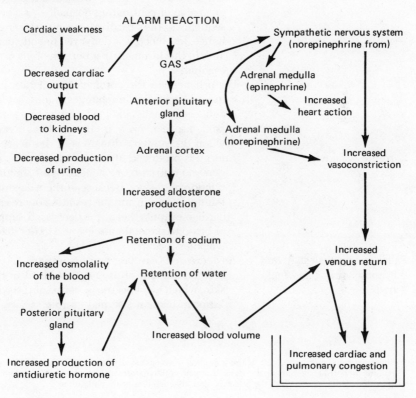

Cardiogenic Shock

215

Let us consider each of Mr. John's signs and symptoms, along with the physiologic explanations, implications, and compensatory mechanisms involved.

Signs and symptoms (what?)	Physiologic explanations (why?) and compensatory mechanisms
	Feeling chilly and apprehensive about being late for his appointment, being unaccustomed to lifting heavy objects, and being angry are stressors that probably precipitated Mr. John's heart attack. Indeed, any one of these stressors could have induced his attack.
Sudden severe pain in the substernal and upper abdominal regions.*	A lack of blood to any part of the body causes pain in that part. The occlusion of a branch of his left coronary artery resulted in decreased flow of blood to his left myocardium. Deprived of sufficient blood, the left myocardium became extremely weak and therefore incapable of contracting normally. As a consequence, the cardiac output declined; hence, less blood was delivered to body parts and, in this instance, to a portion of his myocardium. Disturbances in the coronary circulation frequently lead to reflex changes in muscle tone and, occasionally, in blood supply; therefore, pain also can arise in the skeletal tissues when the primary disease is in the heart.
Extreme weakness.	Energy is produced at the cellular level; oxygen and nutrients are necessary for the production of energy. Because of the weakened left myocardium and the resulting decreased cardiac output, there is a decreased supply of blood to skeletal muscles, and generalized weakness occurs.
Pallor (ashen gray skin) and cyanosis of lips and nail beds.	A decreased cardiac output implies a decreased amount of oxygenated blood to the skin, which would cause ischemia of the skin. Vasoconstriction also plays a role.

* Pain may or may not be present. If the infarction develops slowly, pain may be absent. Ten per cent of the myocardial infarction patients have no pain or discomfort whatever. Because of abdominal pain (with or without vomiting), the attack is often diagnosed as acute indigestion.

Signs and symptoms (what?)	Physiologic explanations (why?) and compensatory mechanisms

	Color of skin
Fast flow of blood through dilated vessels	Scarlet
Slow flow of blood through dilated vessels	Deep blue
Fast flow of blood through constricted vessels	Light pink
Slow flow of blood through constricted vessels	Ashen

Unconsciousness.

A lack of oxygen to the brain causes unconsciousness because brain tissue, in order to function properly, requires a constant supply of oxygen and nutrients (glucose). Obviously, something occurred that prevented a sufficient flow of blood to the brain to maintain a state of consciousness. As the left coronary artery branch became suddenly obstructed, the left ventricular contractions became markedly decreased, arrhythmic, and inadequate; hence, ejection of blood from the left ventricle into the aorta was markedly decreased. Because of the decreased ability of the heart to pump blood, the cardiac output was seriously reduced. Among other things, decreased cardiac output results in a decreased flow of blood through the carotid and vertebral arteries which supply the brain with blood. As a consequence, unconsciousness developed.

In health, a considerable amount of coronary blood flow occurs during diastole, and the flow of blood through the coronary fibers of the inner part of the left ventricle tends to be shut off during systole. In health, when cardiac work is increased, coronary blood flow increases, as does myocardial consumption of oxygen. Mr. John's increased myocardial needs for oxygen were not met, because his obstructed coronary vessel prevented a sufficient flow of blood into part of his left myocardium in the ventricular area. The left ventricular contractions, as a consequence, became weak and insufficient to meet the imminent needs of the left myocardium.

On arrival at the hospital, semiconscious and confused.

Mr. John was transported to the hospital in a supine position. The driver had loosened his necktie and collar. The effects of gravity and

Signs and symptoms (what?)	Physiologic explanations (why?) and compensatory mechanisms
	the removal of any constriction around his neck had increased the flow of blood to his brain, thus returning him to a state of semi-consciousness; however, the blood flow was insufficient to restore full mental faculties;
Severe dyspnea and increased respiratory rate.	thus, the patient was confused. "Dyspnea" means labored breathing. Dyspnea results when the tidal-volume–vital-capacity ratio increases. The normal ratio is 1:9. In congestive heart failure, the accumulation of fluid in the lungs diminishes the vital capacity, and the tidal volume is usually increased. Therefore, elevated tidal volume and decreased vital capacity change the ratio so that it may be 1:3. The pooling of blood in
PWP = 24 mm. Hg. CVP = 18 cm. H$_2$O (increased).	the lungs activates the pressoreceptors in the pulmonary vessels, and the resulting impulses are propagated to the respiratory center to increase the rate of respiration. Due to the inability of the heart muscle to pump adequately, blood that is not forced out of the left ventricle will dam up into the pulmonary circuit, causing engorgement and, eventually, a perfusion of plasma into the alveoli. The alveolar surface area for diffusion of gases is thus greatly reduced, and severe dyspnea results. Also, the small amount of oxygen that does diffuse across the unfilled portions of the alveoli cannot be delivered adequately, owing to the decreased pumping action of the heart. Carbon dioxide, unable to diffuse out of the pulmonary blood stream, accumulates and mixes with the arterial blood, causing hypercapnia. This increased carbon dioxide stimulates the respiratory center in the medulla oblongata of the brain, which raises the respiratory rate. Rales may or may not be heard in the chest. Severe congestion is usually accompanied by wet breathing.

A compensatory shift of blood from the peripheral vessels to the heart occurred in Mr. John as a result of sympathetic nervous system stimulation and the release of norepineph-

Signs and symptoms (what?)	Physiologic explanations (why?) and compensatory mechanisms
Increased pallor.	rine from the adrenal medullae, the effects of which caused peripheral vasoconstriction. Although this compensatory mechanism increases the venous return of blood with the primary purpose of increasing the cardiac output, it can also exaggerate the cardiac and pulmonary congestion, and it often does, especially if the right heart is functioning normally. A distinction should be made between the compensatory mechanisms in moderate (compensated) heart failure and those in severe (decompensated) heart failure. The following mechanisms are involved: *Autonomic reflexes* Strong stimulation from the sympathetic nervous system increases the strength of the heart pump, often as much as 100 per cent. Also, initial peripheral vasoconstriction increases the venous return and the arterial blood pressure. In a less severe heart failure, this increased venous return primes the heart pump, which in turn causes an increased cardiac output. In severe left heart
BP = 110/50. M.A.P. = 70 mm. Hg.	failure, however, this increased venous return of blood will accumulate in the pulmonary circuit, because the left ventricle is too weak to pump it into the systemic circulation.
↓GFR Oliguria.	*Renal retention of fluid* Decreased cardiac output causes a decreased flow of blood to the kidneys; hence, renal functioning is decreased because of the decreased blood pressure and the decreased glomerular filtration pressure in the kidneys. Because of the increased sympathetic stimulation the afferent arterioles of the kidneys become markedly constricted; therefore, glomerular pressure, and the glomerular filtration rate are reduced even more. Thus, with the retention of fluid by the kidneys, the blood volume increases. This increased blood volume, in moderate heart attacks, serves as a beneficial prime to the heart.

Signs and symptoms (what?)	Physiologic explanations (why?) and compensatory mechanisms
	Sodium and fluid retention
	The heart attack sets off the alarm reaction in the body, and the adrenal cortical glands secrete large amounts of aldosterone. The aldosterone causes the retention of sodium, which, in turn, retains water in the body. This water retention causes an increase in the extracellular fluid and the blood volume; hence, venous return is increased.
	Stimulation of the antidiuretic hormone
	The increased retention of sodium increases the osmotic concentration (osmolality) of the extracellular fluid. This increased osmolality elicits an increased secretion of the antidiuretic hormone (ADH) from the posterior pituitary gland. ADH, in turn, promotes a further retention of water in the body.
Pulse rapid, irregular, and very weak.	The beat of the heart is reflected in the pulse. Cardiac contractions are very weak and arrhythmic, owing to the decreased strength to the left myocardium. Ventricular fibrillation is often present. Defibrillation is indicated immediately.
Decreased blood pressure: BP = 90/40. M.A.P. = 57.	The decreased heart action resulting in a decreased cardiac output of blood is the cause of the low blood pressure. Later, peripheral vasodilatation would accentuate the low blood pressure.
Anuria.	If the cardiac output is less than normal, i.e., if it falls to as low as one half to two thirds of normal, anuria is likely to result. In general, the urinary output will be less than normal if the cardiac output is less than normal. Five liters of cardiac output per minute is required for normal renal function. Patients
Unconscious.	with severe heart attacks sometimes develop sudden severe pulmonary edema a week or so after the acute attack and die a respiratory death (rather than a death resulting from a diminished cardiac output) due to reduced renal function, i.e., sufficient fluid is retained to overload the circulatory system.

PHYSIOLOGICAL PRINCIPLES IN THE TREATMENT
OF PATIENTS IN HEART FAILURE

Rational treatment is dependent on the effectiveness of an action to reverse altered physiology. The principles in the management of patients with heart failure are:

"reduce cardiac demand
improve cardiac performance
maximize the rate and completeness of healing
reverse associated disorders of organ function
and fluid balance."[2]

MEDICAL MANAGEMENT

Over the past 15 to 20 years, vasopressor drugs were the mainstay of treatment of myocardial infarction patients in cardiogenic shock. Limited benefits obtained from vasopressor therapy led to a search for better forms of treatment. Subsequently, this led to the use of vasodilator drugs. According to Binder and Shubin, "Therapy has been a matter of vogue, rather than a fundamental understanding of the natural history of this condition."[3]

Presently, vasodilators are in vogue; a chief one being sodium nitroprusside. Although vasodilators decrease the arterial resistance; hence, decreasing the resistance to cardiac output, they can also reduce coronary perfusion pressure, which adds insult to injury in an already ischemic myocardium. Yet, until the advent of the aortic counterpulsation balloon (also called intra-aortic balloon pump, or IABP) which augments coronary blood flow, and myocardial revascularization surgery, the mortality rate remained high. It will be interesting to see what posterity holds for the treatment of patients in cardiogenic shock.

INTRA-AORTIC BALLOON PUMP (IABP)

To support patients in cardiogenic shock, an intra-aortic balloon is positioned in the descending thoracic aorta just distal to the left

[2] H. J. C. Swan and W. W. Parmley. "Congestive Heart Failure," in *Pathologic Physiology*, 5th ed. (William A. Sodeman and William A. Sodeman, Jr., Eds.), Philadelphia: W. B. Saunders Co., 1974, p. 290.
[3] Maxwell Binder and Herbert Shubin. "Shock Due to Myocardial Infarction," in *Shock: Diagnosis and Treatment*, Baltimore: Williams and Wilkins Co., 1967, p. 144.

subclavian artery. (It is inserted in the femoral artery and threaded through the abdominal aorta.) In synchrony with the mechanical events of the heart, the balloon is inflated and deflated. On systole, the balloon deflates, and on diastole it inflates. Normally, the systolic contraction of the heart forces blood into the coronary artery. On diastole, in health, the blood is emptied from the coronary artery into the myocardium. Therefore, since the balloon inflates on diastole, more blood is diverted from the aorta into the coronary artery, thus augmenting coronary blood flow. A pressing problem is the difficulty of weaning the patients off of the balloon.

Recently, Dr. William S. Pierce of the Pennsylvania State University, reported on a pneumatically powered, paracorporeal, pulsatile assist pump that may provide a more satisfactory and reliable support of heart function in open heart surgery patients than the intra-aortic balloon pump. The device lies alongside the patient, and can be removed under local anesthesia.[4]

EXTERNAL COUNTERPULSATION FOR CARDIOGENIC SHOCK

According to Begley, external counter-pulsation (ECP) increases the diastolic pressure and decreases the systolic pressure, and has been successful in treating patients in cardiogenic shock. Each leg, from ankle to thigh, is inserted into a rigid cylinder. A water-filled bag fills the space between the leg and cylinder. Water is pumped in and out of the bag, exerting a uniform pressure over the surface of the legs and on the arteries and veins. On diastole of the heart, a positive pressure is applied that increases myocardial perfusion. Negative pressure, on systole of the heart, aspirates blood out of the heart. Each treatment period is approximately three hours.[5]

REVASCULARIZATION SURGERY

The saphenous vein is presently used as a bypass around the occluded coronary artery, thus providing an increased amount of blood to the myocardial muscle. The intra-aortic balloon pump is usually used in conjunction with surgery.

---

[4] "Paracorporeal Pump Provides Prolonged Circulatory Support," *Hospital Practice* (March 1978), 40–43.
[5] Linda A. Begley. "External Counterpulsation for Cardiogenic Shock," *American Journal of Nursing*, 75 (June 1975), 967–970.

Nursing Care of the Patient in Cardiogenic Shock

Mr. John is in shock, not because of a decreased blood volume and not because of an increase in the size of the vascular bed, but because of an inefficient cardiac muscle pump which cannot force the blood through the arterial circulatory circuit. The result, of course, is the same as the result of other types of shock—decreased blood to the body tissues resulting in tissue hypoxia. With a damming up of blood in the left atrium and ventricle and in the pulmonary venous circuit, pulmonary congestion occurs. Subsequently, pulmonary hypoxia and marked dyspnea become manifest. Cyanosis, in this instance, is due not to a decreased amount of hemoglobin (as it is in hemorrhagic shock), but to the reduced hemoglobin in the red blood cells. The hemoglobin is reduced (lacks oxygen) because of the poor diffusion of oxygen from the alveoli into the pulmonary capillary blood stream.

Quick action and proper nursing care are indicated for the patient in cardiogenic shock. Only the combined and integrated actions of the nurse-doctor team offer hope for saving the patient's life. The nurse's activities should be purposeful and based on a scientific background. Major nursing measures include:

1. Proper patient-positioning
2. Relief of pain and apprehension
3. Monitoring of vital signs, noting comparative changes in the heart rate, blood pressure, electrocardiogram, central venous pressure, and pulmonary wedge pressure
4. Measurement of output every 15–30 minutes
5. Administration of drugs
6. Administration of oxygen with pressure or volume-controlled ventilators
7. Suctioning, PRN
8. Assessing level of consciousness
9. Direct observation of patient: skin color, temperature, clamminess
10. Decreasing metabolic needs to decrease cardiac burden
11. In the absence of a physician, defibrillation to establish a normal sinus rhythm (if the heart is in ventricular fibrillation).

Scientific rationale will be presented in the following pages.

OBJECTIVES AND PRINCIPLES OF NURSING CARE

What is needed is intelligent action based on proper objectives and principles that the nurse has formulated, or is formulating, in her mind. It is the registered nurse who calls the signals to mobilize her nursing forces for purposeful action. If she has been accustomed to think in terms of objectives and to qualify them with principles, she will have little difficulty in formulating a pattern of care. Of prime importance is that the most important objectives be given priority over all other objectives; first things first. The ability to make quick, accurate decisions increases with professional growth and practice.

OBJECTIVE 1: Provide for an increased circulation of blood to the brain.

PRINCIPLE 52: A constant supply of oxygen and nutrients is requisite for the life and proper functioning of brain tissue.

BODY POSITION

Due to the weakness of Mr. John's heart, the output of blood into the arterial circuit is markedly decreased; hence, the quantity of blood to the brain via the carotid and vertebral arteries is decreased. From her observance of signs such as semiconsciousness and confusion, the nurse knows that blood in sufficient quantity and/or quality is not reaching the brain. Therefore, she places the patient in a supine position, so that blood, without the resistance of gravity, can flow more freely to the brain. If he is conscious, a low Fowler's position is indicated to ensure better oxygenation of the brain. Let us trace the logic of this. In a low Fowler's position (1) the diaphragm is somewhat lower which aids the respiratory excursion and provides more room for pulmonary expansion; hence, more alveolar surface area is available for the diffusion of oxygen and carbon dioxide. The oxygenation of the blood is therefore increased. (2) The slight degree of gravity favors pulmonary venous emptying into the left atrium which tends to relieve the congestion in the pulmonary circuit. (3) There is less resistance to the return of venous blood from the brain via the superior vena cava to the right atrium; hence, stagnant anoxia of the brain tissues is prevented. For unconsciousness, however, a supine position is indicated.

224

OBJECTIVE 2:   Provide for an adequate exchange of respiratory gases. Provide for increased pulmonary diffusion of oxygen and carbon dioxide.

PRINCIPLE 36:   The passage of oxygen from the atmosphere to the lungs and the passage of carbon dioxide from the blood stream to the atmosphere are dependent on an open airway.

PRINCIPLE 53:   For the diffusion of a gas across a membrane, direct contact of the gas with the membrane is requisite.

PRINCIPLE 9:   The amount of gas that can diffuse across a membrane is proportionate to the quantity and partial pressure of the gas and the circumference of the surface area of the membrane with which the gas is in direct contact.

PRINCIPLE 34:   Fluids and gases flow from greater to lesser points of pressure.

Thus it can be seen that Objectives 1 and 2 are closely intertwined. An increased amount of poorly oxygenated blood to the brain would have little or no beneficial effect on the brain cells. Therefore, it is imperative that every effort is made to ensure increased oxygenation of the pulmonary blood stream. Immediate follow-up treatment including the administration of oxygen and digitalis (as ordered) will strengthen myocardial contractions thus dramatically improving both the respiratory status and the circulation of oxygenated blood to the brain.

A fourth reason to justify a low Fowler's position to improve the circulatory-respiratory status of the patient is that in a low Fowler's position, the return of venous blood from the lower part of the body to the right atrium would be decreased. While this decreased return may seem negligible, it certainly does not favor an increased accumulation of blood in the pulmonary circuit (review pulmonary circulation).* As a matter of fact, the use of tourniquets (which may be ordered) on three extremities is for the purpose of decreasing the right atrial inflow load, thereby relieving the pulmonary circuit. At any rate, proper positioning of the patient with severe heart failure is an important factor which affects circulation and respiration.

---

* Pulmonary circulation: On cardiac systole, venous blood is forced from the right ventricle into the pulmonary artery (which divides into right and left branches) and is delivered to the lungs. Carbon dioxide leaves the venous blood by diffusing into the respiratory tract, while oxygen from the respiratory tract diffuses into the same blood stream. This oxygenated blood (referred to as arterial blood) is then delivered, via the four pulmonary veins, to the left atrium.

Left heart failure is characterized by severe dyspnea and pulmonary edema. Cyanosis is often present, also. It is not always possible for the nurse to know the patient's diagnosis when he is admitted. It is at times such as this that she must rely on her professional observations, judgment, and ingenuity to save a life. A physician may, or may not be present when such a patient is brought to the hospital. For this reason, the nurse must function expeditiously on her own until a physician arrives.

Dyspnea and cyanosis are obvious clues of oxygen deficiency, and the administration of oxygen is vital for this patient. Cyanosis, the nurse reasons, is the result of decreased oxygen in the hemoglobin of the red blood cells. Either oxygen isn't entering the hemoglobin in sufficient quantities, or the quantity of hemoglobin is insufficient to carry the oxygen. In either case, the administration of oxygen is justified. While Mr. John has sufficient hemoglobin to carry oxygen, the amount of oxygen diffusing across the pulmonary alveolar membranes is decreased because of his pulmonary congestion. Although the hemoglobin and the volume of blood are sufficient, pallor and cyanosis appear because the blood is not being pumped adequately through the circulatory circuit.

Some physicians prefer oxygen given with a positive-pressure apparatus. The force of the positive pressure aids in the alveolar expansion and the diffusion of oxygen, so that the hemoglobin in the pulmonary blood stream becomes better saturated with oxygen. Before oxygen is given, however, the nurse should make sure that the upper respiratory passages are clear of any mucus that could prevent the passage of oxygen to the lower respiratory passages. Noisy breathing indicates such an obstruction. However, this should not be relied on solely in determining whether such an obstruction is present. Many times an obstruction exists in the absence of noisy breath sounds. For this reason, the nurse should use the oronasal suction apparatus. It takes such a little time to make sure that the upper respiratory passages are clear.

The force by which the oxygen enters the alveoli with the use of a positive-pressure machine will tend to be greater than the force within the pulmonary capillary blood stream; hence, fluid that has perfused from the blood stream into the alveoli will be pushed from the alveoli back into the blood stream. Despite the fact that the cardiac output is greatly diminished, what little blood it does put into the arterial circuit will be more heavily laden with oxygen. The oxygen, along with a supine position (if the patient is unconscious) will provide for a better circulation of oxygenated blood to the brain. Also, although the blood supply to the myocardium is insufficient in quantity, the amount of oxygen to it will be greatly increased; thus, myocardial strength will tend to increase.

The physiologic basis for cardiac dyspnea is an increased pulmonary venous pressure. Any measure that can successfully lower this pressure can be expected to lessen respiratory distress. Morphine is the most useful drug in treating patients with acute pulmonary edema. It is not known how morphine promptly reverses acute pulmonary edema; however, it is postulated that it may be related to the interruption of reflex arcs set up by the rising venous pressure.

OBJECTIVE 3: Relieve pain.
PRINCIPLE 54: Splinting of a painful area of the body is a protective measure to prevent further pain.
SUBPRINCIPLES   a. Severe pain in the chest area is accompanied by decreased motion of the respiratory musculature.

b. Decreased motion of the respiratory musculature implies a decreased vital capacity, hence, decreased alveolar expansion, decreased intake of oxygen, and decreased output of carbon dioxide.

c. Pain increases apprehension which, in turn, increases the cardiac burden.

d. The absence of pain in an area is accompanied by a freer, more normal motion of that area.

Respiratory insufficiency is one of the major problems of the patient who has a left myocardial infarction. For this reason, concerted effort must be made to relieve the patient of respiratory distress. Because severe anginal chest pain decreases respiratory excursions, it is logical to relieve the patient of pain as quickly as possible. Opiates, such as morphine or codeine, are usually ordered and should be given at once. Nitroglycerine under the tongue or inhalation of amyl nitrate also helps to relieve the pain.

Splinting of the painful chest is accompanied by rapid, shallow respirations; hence, the inhaled air reaches the alveoli under a very low pressure, a pressure that is incapable of forcing the abnormal plasma fluid in the alveoli back into the pulmonary capillary blood stream. Pulmonary edema and, hence, dyspnea persist. After the administration of a narcotic, however, the respirations become slower and deeper. Unless the patient is relieved of his pain, his condition can only become worse.

Many physicians advocate that opiates and barbiturate sedatives be given around the clock for the first week. The relief of the patient's pain, anxiety, and activity afforded by these drugs, it is felt, far outweighs the disadvantages of a depressed cough reflex.

OBJECTIVE 4: Provide for adequate circulation of blood to the myocardium.

OBJECTIVE 55: A constant supply of oxygen, nutrients, fluid, electrolytes, and hormones (blood), and the removal of wastes from the myocardium are basic for adequate myocardial contractions.

Nitroglycerine tablets, in small repeated doses, are usually ordered to be placed under the patient's tongue to dissolve there. This drug dilates the coronary arteries, thus providing for increased circulation of blood to the myocardium. Also, it favors the development of a collateral circulation in the myocardium and tends to limit the size of the infarct. The patient is usually permitted to have a supply of nitroglycerine tablets at his bedside, to be taken as needed. Isordil may also be ordered.

Assist the physician with the insertion of an aortic counterpulsation balloon. This augments coronary blood flow, thereby increasing myocardial perfusion.

PRINCIPLE 56: An adequate flow of blood through the arterial circuit (including the coronary arteries) is dependent on an adequate pump to propel it.

OBJECTIVE 5: Provide for an increased cardiac output. Provide for increased strength of myocardial contractions.

PRINCIPLE 57: If all other factors remain constant, cardiac output is proportionate to the strength of myocardial contractions.

A beta-adrenergic blocking drug, such as Inderal, may be ordered for cardiac arrhythmias. This drug lessens the intense stimulation of the heart due to epinephrine and norepinephrine.

PRINCIPLE 15: An adequate cardiac output is basic to the health and proper functioning of all body tissues.

Thus far, the nurse has taken steps to provide for increased circulation of blood to the brain, increased oxygenation of the pulmonary blood stream, and the relief of the patient's pain. These are all important objectives; however, the achievement of these objectives without providing for the increased strength and output of the heart would be useless.

228

One of the most important objectives, medically, is to establish a cardiac rhythm, rate, and output which are compatible with life.

Digitalis is often the drug of choice to achieve this objective. Digitalis decreases the heart rate and strengthens myocardial contractions, resulting in an increased cardiac output. For quick results, the physician may administer the drug intravenously.* Presently, opinions differ as to the efficacy of digitalis. It is the concensus that digitalis should be withheld until decreased potassium is corrected.

A bolus dose of a corticosteroid to improve the chronotropic effects of the heart is often administered. By improving cardiac output, the amount of blood going through the coronary arteries is greater.

The patient should be kept at *complete* bed rest. All of his needs should be taken care of by the nurse. Any effort on the part of the patient would increase his metabolic needs, and therefore increase the needs of the myocardium for more blood.

By strengthening cardiac contractions and decreasing cardiac rate, several important results will be achieved: (1) the cardiac output will be increased; (2) the left ventricular-atrial-pulmonary-venous high-pressure dam will be relieved, and the blood in the left circuit will resume a more normal flow through the systemic arterial circuit; (3) the pressure within the pulmonary capillary blood stream will decrease considerably, with a subsequent discouragement of perfusion of plasma fluid into the pulmonary alveoli—there is a subsiding of fluid from the alveoli back into the capillary blood stream; (4) the myocardium will receive a greater quantity of oxygenated blood; and (5) all tissues of the body will receive greater amounts of blood.

As the patient becomes properly digitalized, one notices a disappearance of his signs and symptoms. The results are dramatic: with the improvement of the cardiocirculatory status, the cyanosis and pallor disappear, the skin becomes warm and dry, the dypsnea subsides, the mental faculties become clearer, the pulse becomes stronger and more regular, and the blood pressure rises.

OBJECTIVE 6:   Relieve cardiac burden. Provide for increased urinary output.
PRINCIPLE 58:   An increase in circulating fluid volume increases the heart's workload.

---

* Observe patient for signs of digitalis toxicity: depression, nausea and vomiting, and disturbances of heart rhythm.

The mechanisms affecting the retention of fluids have been discussed (aldosterone and the antidiuretic hormone). The greatly increased volume of circulating fluids can be decreased by several means:

1. Digitalis. Although digitalis is not a true diuretic, it has diuretic affects in that by strengthening cardiac contractions and increasing the cardiac output more blood is forced into the afferent arteries of the kidneys; hence, the glomerular filtration pressure is raised, and the production of urine is increased.

2. A decreased intake—restriction of fluids.

3. Decreased salt in the diet lowers the concentration of the extracellular fluids, and increased renal output follows.

4. Administration of diuretics brings about a balance between fluid intake and output, despite a low cardiac output.

Occasionally, cardiac shock is treated by intravenous administration of blood, plasma, or other fluids, in an effort to prime the heart like a pump and thus increase the cardiac output. This is not practical, however, if the patient has serious pulmonary edema. Extra fluids administered to such a patient could actually drown him. He should be observed for dyspnea, basal rales, and neck vein distention—all of which are signs of an overloaded circulatory circuit that the weakened heart cannot handle.

In the absence of acute pulmonary edema, a colloid solution may be ordered to offset the increased hydrostatic pressure in the pulmonary interstitium. About 20 per cent of patients with myocardial infarction develop a state of relative hypovolemia which occurs secondary to vasodilatation (after compensatory vasoconstriction failure). This produces an inadequate effective circulating volume. If the CVP, pulmonary wedge pressure, and left ventricular end diastolic pressure are low, intravenous fluids are usually ordered. Such fluids may be 5 per cent glucose in water, dextran, or salt-poor albumin. Heparin is often added to prevent the clotting of the blood.

OBJECTIVE 7: Decrease the metabolic needs of the body.

PRINCIPLE 59: Physical and/or emotional activity increase the metabolic needs of the body.

PRINCIPLE 2: Increased metabolism is accompanied by increased cellular needs for oxygen and nutrients, and increased formation of metabolites.

PRINCIPLE 18: Increased metabolism imples increased demands on cardiac output.

One degree Centigrade elevation of body temperature imposes a 25 per cent extra burden on the heart to pump blood. This is due to the general increased metabolic needs of the body. Therefore, the patient should be kept as cool as possible, without shivering. External heat in any form should *NOT* be applied, unless shivering occurs. (This subject has been covered previously.)

Physical and/or emotional activity of any nature or degree could prove fatal to the patient who is in cardiogenic shock. Since cardiogenic shock represents a crucial inability of the heart to function normally, even when the patient is at complete bed rest, physical and/or emotional stress, causing an increase in body metabolism, would place an additional burden on the heart. For this reason, absolute physical and emotional rest must be maintained from the first moment of our contact with the patient until all his signs and symptoms of danger are ameliorated. Often, the patient is not permitted to turn himself or to sit up. Maximum rest should be provided during the acute stage, and the patient should be disturbed as little as possible during the hours of sleep.

A sedative, such as phenobarbital, is a very useful adjunct in providing for physical relaxation and the relief of mental tension. Sedatives, however, are only adjuncts and should not be relied upon solely to accomplish this important objective.

In a study done by McNeal, it was found that rectal temperatures cause no significant changes in the heart rate of patients with acute myocardial infarctions.[6] No bradycardia occurred. She found that significant heart rate changes occurred during the turning phase. Nursing care implications for this is to teach the patient to turn properly to prevent the Valsalva maneuver, i.e., the patient should turn while taking slow deep breaths with the mouth open.

Anyone coming in contact with the patient—and this includes relatives and other visitors, nursing personnel, doctors, and other hospital staff—has a decided effect on the physical and emotional well-being of the patient. It should be explained to the patient's visitors that lengthy and/or controversial discussions could prove very dangerous to the patient's well-being. Also, the number of visitors and visits should be held at an absolute minimum—at least until the danger period has passed. It must be remembered that visitors do not possess our understanding of the patient's condition, hence, it is not sufficient to

[6] Gloria J. McNeal. "Rectal Temperatures in the Patient with an Acute Myocardial Infarction," *Image*, 10 (Feb. 1978), 18–23.

tell, or even to ask them to restrict their visits and conversations with the patient—we must follow up our request with explanations. Simply telling them that "It is best for the patient," is grossly insufficient; we must explain in simple lay terms the anatomic-physiologic basis for our requests. Nurses who understand the anatomic and physiologic implications usually will not shirk this teaching responsibility.

On the other hand, nurses who do not understand these implications are prone to make such nebulous statements as "The *doctor* wishes it," or "It's a hospital policy"—ridiculous and insufficient statements that do nothing but provoke anger and affect the patient's condition adversely.

Every patient is an individual who reacts in his own way. For this reason, our adjustments and approaches to him must be flexible and patient-centered. We must learn to accept the patient as he is, rather than think that he will behave as we expect. It is not our prerogative to expect the patient to adjust to us, but it is our responsibility to adapt to the patient. This is much easier said than done. A nurse does not become tolerant of others because she has been told to do so. It is not always easy to adapt to patients; indeed, at times it is most difficult because personalities and behaviors are formed from varying hereditary, racial, and environmental backgrounds, and our own backgrounds could be very different from those of many patients. Although our nursing procedures might be above reproach, we must keep a constant inward eye on our attitudes, expressions, and choice of words, or else we might be instrumental in adding to the patient's emotional strain. While we are administering oxygen and medications, while we are checking vital signs, while we are requesting the patient to remain as quiet as possible, our expressions and our voices must be courteous and gentle, and, at times, firmly persuasive. We must realize that the patient does not understand many of our procedures, and many requests we make of him. When indicated, the nurse should sit down and explain to patients, but she should not go into a lengthy discourse until she has completed those tasks that will free the patient of imminent danger. The patient who knows he is very close to death would prefer that we *do* for him rather than talk with him at this crucial time.

The main objectives for the patient in cardiogenic shock have been discussed. These objectives are closely intertwined; for example, by strengthening and slowing the heart rate, the circulation to the brain will be increased, as well as myocardial circulation. By relieving the patient of pain, the exchange of respiratory gases will be improved. The steps toward the accomplishment of one objective, therefore, are related to the accomplishment of other objectives. Or, we might say that it is rare to take care of one need without also taking care of another need.

REFERENCES

Boyd, J. M. "Understanding and Treating Cardiogenic Shock," *RN* (April 1975), 53–62.

Burman, Sheldon O., and Elias O. Decio. "Mechanical and Circulatory Assistance in Shock," in *Treatment of Shock; Principles and Practice* (William Schumer and Lloyd Nyhus, Eds.), Philadelphia: Lea and Febiger, 1974.

Cavanagh, Denis, S. Papineni, S. Rao and M. Comas. *Septic Shock in Obstetrics and Gynecology*, Philadelphia: W. B. Saunders Co., 1977.

Chaffee, Ellen and Esther Greisheimer. *Basic Physiology and Anatomy*, 3rd ed., Philadelphia: J. B. Lippincott Co., 1974.

da Luz, Protasio L., Max H. Weil and Herbert Shubin. "Current Concepts on Mechanisms and Treatment of Cardiogenic Shock," *American Heart Journal*, 92 (Jully 1976), 103–113.

Daniell, Herman B. "Coronary Flow Alterations on Myocardial Contractility, Oxygen Extraction, and Oxygen Consumption," *American Journal of Physiology*, 225 (Nov. 1973), 1020–1025.

Gunnar, Rolf M., Henry Loeb, Sarah Johnson and Patric Scanlon. "Cardiovascular Assist Devices in Cardiogenic Shock," *Journal of the American Medical Association*, 236 (Oct. 4, 1976), 1619–1621.

Guyton, Arthur C. *Textbook of Medical Physiology*, 5th ed., Philadelphia: W. B. Saunders Co., 1976.

Thorne, G., R. Adams, E. Brauwald, K. Isselbacher and R. Petersdorf. Harrison's *Principle's of Internal Medicine*, 8th ed., New York: McGraw-Hill Book Co., 1977.

Langley, L. L. *Reveiw of Physiology*, 3rd ed., New York: McGraw-Hill Book Co., 1971.

McCredie, John A. (Ed.). *Basic Surgery*, New York: Macmillan Publishing Co., Inc., 1977.

Mehta, Jawahar. "Vasodilators in the Treatment of Heart Failure," *Journal of the American Medical Association*, 238 (Dec. 5, 1977), 2534–2536.

Resnekov, Leon. "Management of Acute Myocardial Infarction," *Cardiovascular Medicine*, 2 (Oct. 1977), 949–956.

Shires, G. Tom (Ed.). *Care of the Trauma Patient*, New York: McGraw-Hill Book Co., 1966.

Siegel, John H. "The Heart in Shock, in *Treatment of Shock: Principles and Practice* (William Schumer and Lloyd Nyhus, eds.), Philadelphia: Lea and Febiger, 1974, pp. 104–121.

Sodeman, William, and William Sodeman, Jr. *Pathologic Physiology*, 5th ed., Philadelphia: W. B. Saunders Co., 1974.

Swan, H. J. C., J. S. Forrester, G. Diamond, K. Chatterje and W. W. Parmley. "Hemodynamic Spectrum of Myocardial Infarction and Cardiogenic Shock," *Circulation*, 1972, 1097–1110.

Thal, Alan P., E. B. Brown, Jr., Arlo S. Hermreck and Hugh H. Bell. *Shock: A Physiologic Basis for Treatment*, Chicago: Year Book Medical Publishers, 1971.

Weil, Max H. and Herbert Shubin. *Diagnosis and Treatment of Shock*, Baltimore: Williams and Wilkins Co., 1967.

Winkle, Roger and D. Harrison. "Beta Blockers in the Treatment of Acute Arrhythmias," *Heart and Lung*, 6 (Jan.–Feb. 1977), 62–67.

Ziesche, Susan and Joseph Franciosa. "Clinical Application of Sodium Nitroprusside," *Heart and Lung*, 6 (Jan.–Feb. 1977), 99–103.

CHAPTER 11

Shock Due to Chest Injuries

Shock caused by chest injuries is more often the result of deranged cardiorespiratory function than of blood loss.

Normal Anatomy of the Lungs*

Normally, the pressure between the visceral and parietal pleurae is negative. It is this negative pressure that maintains the lung in an expanded state. If the negative pressure is destroyed, such as by a tear in either the visceral or parietal pleura, then positive air (the same as the atmospheric air we breathe) will rush in and destroy the negative pressure and create an actual pleural space. With the entrance of positive pressure creating a pleural space, there is a relative collapse of the lung.

PRINCIPLE 34.   Gases flow from greater to lesser points of pressure.

* Note: For diagrammatic purposes, the visceral and parietal pleurae are shown in Fig. 24. Normally, they fit closely, like a glove on a hand.

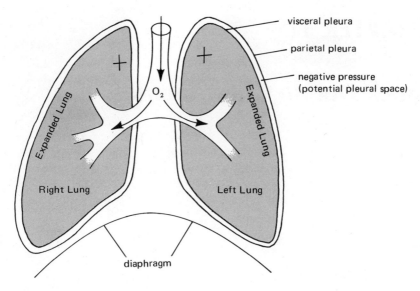

Figure 24. *Normal lungs.*

Closed Tension Pneumothorax

Dr. A. P. Carney III was driving to his animal hospital. All of a sudden, he sneezed violently. Immediately he pulled up at the curb and stopped the car. Gasping for air, he clutched his right chest in pain. "My God," he moaned, "It's happened again. . . . I've had a spontaneous pneumothorax." Apprehensively, he deliberated, and deciding that he could make it to the hospital a quarter of a mile away, he started the car and took off.

Upon arrival at the emergency room, he told the triage nurse that he thought he had a collapsed lung; the same as he had had two years previously. Dr. Carney was dizzy, apprehensive, weak, cyanotic, and dyspneic.

Immediately the nurse contacted a physician and told him what had happened. Treatment was instituted immediately. The nurse administered an analgesic for pain, and the physician inserted a thoracotomy tube into the pleural space and connected the other end to an underwater sealed drainage bottle. Within a half hour, Dr. Carney's color had improved, his apprehension and dizziness disappeared, he felt stronger, and he was breathing normally.

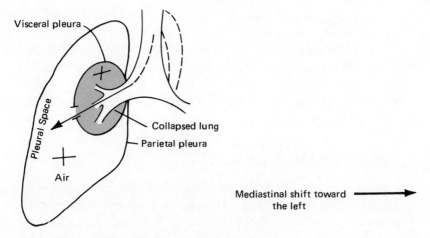

Visceral pleura

Pleural Space

Collapsed lung

Parietal pleura

Air

Mediastinal shift toward the left →

Figure 25. *Closed tension pneumothorax.*

Figure 26. *Thoractomy tube inserted into the pleural space. Tube is connected to under-water sealed drainage. Pressure in pleural space is thus relieved.*

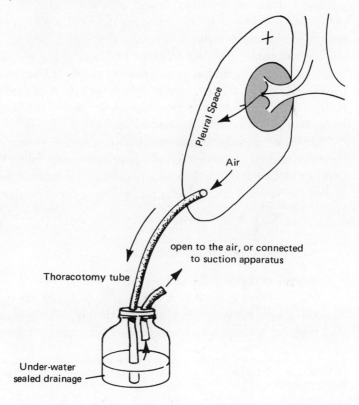

Pleural Space

Air

open to the air, or connected to suction apparatus

Thoracotomy tube

Under-water sealed drainage

The physician stayed with him and said, "It's a good thing you got here when you did. You had a closed tension pneumothorax. We'll take an x-ray and have to take you to surgery to suture the leak in your visceral pleura. And while we're at it, we'll do a poudrage so this won't happen again."

TENSION PNEUMOTHORAX

Dr. Carney had a history of emphysemetous blebs, or bullae, on his right visceral pleura. These weakened areas burst when he sneezed violently, causing the positive pressure in the lung to escape through, thus creating an actual pleural space. Consequently, the right lung collapsed. At the point of the visceral tear, a one-way ball-valve action was produced. On inspiration the valve opened and permitted air to enter the pleural space. On expiration, the valve, or flap, closed over the leak; thus a high pressure built up in the pleural space.

The mediastinum shifted toward the unaffected left lung* thus putting a strain on the inferior and superior venae cavae. As a result of this embarrassment to the venae cavae, there was a decreased venous return to the right atrium; hence, a decreased cardiac output from the left ventricle. Also, his trachea deviated to the left side. Cyanosis dyspnea, dizziness, and apprehension resulted. If Dr. Carney's pleural pressure had not been relieved by the insertion of the thoracotomy tube, with the connection to under-water sealed drainage, he would have died of asphyxia and cerebral hypoxia.

In cases of tension pneumothorax, surgery is required to suture the visceral leak, in order for the lung to expand fully. The presence of other blebs might necessitate a poudrage, i.e., a substance is inserted to seal the visceral and parietal pleurae to prevent recurrent pneumothoraces.

NURSING CARE OF DR. CARNEY

A sealed water drainage

As fluid and gases flow from greater to lesser points of pressure, the only way to rid the pleural space of the air and any pleural drainage that may be present is to connect the thoracotomy tube to an under-

---

* In a pneumothorax without a one-way valve mechanism, the mediastinal shift will be *toward* the affected side. This is due to the equalization of intrapleural and intrapulmonary pressures.

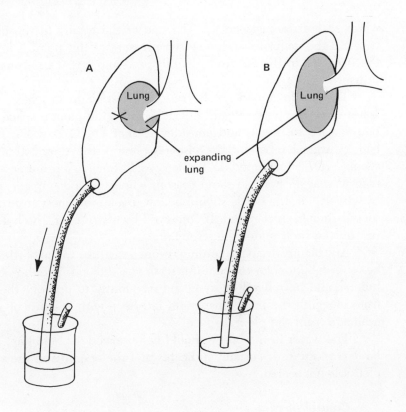

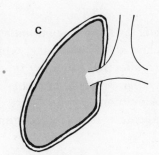

Figure 27. *Re-expansion of the lung.*
  A. *The air leak has been sutured.*
  B. *The lung starts to expand.*
  C. *The lung has expanded, and the thoractomy tube has been removed.*

239

water sealed drainage bottle. The end of the tubing in the bottle is beneath the water level, hence the pressure at this point is less than the pressure in the affected pleural space and less than atmospheric pressure.

The bottle should not be raised higher than the chest, or else water from the bottle would be sucked into the pleural space. If the bottle were to break (and considering that Dr. Carney has not yet had a surgical repair of the visceral pleura), the thoracotomy tube should *NOT* be clamped, as tension would once again increase in his pleural space.* For the same reason, when transporting the patient by wheelchair, the bottle should be lower than the chest and the tube should remain unclamped. If conveyed by a stretcher, the bottle can rest on the shelf under the stretcher.

Any bloody drainage coming through the tube to the bottle should be observed for color to see if it is fresh or old blood. The thoracotomy tube should be milked or squeezed frequently to prevent the blood from clogging the line. This would interfere with the exit of air and drainage from the pleural space.

The water in the bottle should be observed for bubbling. If bubbling continues, this usually indicates that the opening on the visceral pleura is not sealed.

Control of pain

If possible, opiates should be avoided, as these depress ventilation and the cough reflex.

Prevention of atelectasis and pneumonitis

Supporting the chest (front and back) while the patient coughs will provide for a more effective cough by splinting the painful area. If the cough is ineffectual, tracheal-bronchial suctioning should be done. The presence of pulmonary rales, increased pulse and respirations, and dyspnea indicate a need for coughing and/or suctioning.

Questions

1. What was Dr. Carney's probable pulse rate before he was treated? Explain.
2. What caused his cyanosis? (His blood volume was normal.)

* Typically, after surgery, and in the absence of any broncho-pleural fistula, if the bottle breaks, the tubing *should* be clamped in order to prevent a recollapse of the lung. A sterile bottle with sterile water should be secured immediately.

3. Why was he dizzy and apprehensive?
4. In all probability he was oliguric. Explain.
5. If his normal blood pressure was 120/80:
    a. Would his systolic pressure be higher or lower before he was treated? Explain.
    b. Would his diastolic pressure be higher or lower before he was treated? Explain.
    c. What are the implications on his coronary blood flow?
6. How did the General Adaptation Syndrome help him?
7. Why would it *not* be correct to clamp Dr. Carney's thoracotomy tube (before surgery) if his bottle were to break?

Open Pneumothorax (Sucking Wound)

An open pneumothorax means that air enters from the outside, destroys the negative pressure between the visceral and parietal pleurae, and thus creates a pleural space. Causes of an open pneumothorax are penetrating wounds, such as stab wounds.

As air enters and creates a pleural space, the mediastinum shifts back and forth (the Pendlelluft phenomenon). This shift causes the shift of stale air from one lung to the other, resulting in a relative state of asphyxia. There is a decreased venous return which results in a decreased cardiac output. Circulatory shock can ensue if not treated.

Figure 28. *Open pneumothorax.*

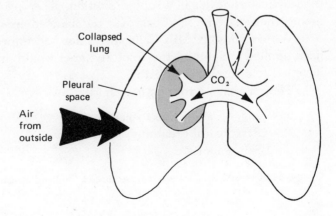

EMERGENCY TREATMENT OF OPEN PNEUMOTHORAX

Emergency treatment entails covering and sealing the external wound to prevent the further admission of air into the pleural space. Preferably, an air-tight dressing with the use of vaseline gauze, should be used. If this is not possible, the hand should seal the wound.

As soon as possible, a thoracotomy tube should be inserted into the pleural space (by a physician), and connected to an under-water sealed drainage bottle to enable the re-expansion of the lung. If this bottle were to break (remember, the air has entered from the outside, and *not* from the lung), the tube should be clamped immediately.

Shock Due to Multiple Rib-Fractures

Normal respiratory function is dependent upon the integrity of the rib cage, pleura, and lungs.

RIB FRACTURES

Miss Ardelle Callahan was standing on the uppermost rung of a ladder as she sawed dead limbs from a tree. Losing her balance, Miss Callahan fell to the ground. Immediately she moaned with pain as she tried to sit up. Joe, her next door neighbor, rushed to her and saw that her color was pale and that she was obviously short of breath. He helped her to his car and drove to the nearest emergency room. By this time, Miss Callahan was extremely restless, and wild-eyed. Her skin color was very pale and her nail beds and lips were cyanotic. Joe told the attending physician what had happened. Immediately the physician put her in a supine position, observed her chest movements, then placed a sand bag over the affected area.

Within minutes, Miss Callahan's color had improved. Failure to have applied weight* to the fractured area would, in all probability, have led to a respiratory death.

The physician wrote on her chart:

5:00 P.M. on admission to E.R.:
    Paradoxical breathing; left flail chest
    Skin pallor

---

* *Any* type of weight is indicated, the pressure of the hand or fist, a brick, and so on.

Cyanosis of nail beds and lips

Extremely agitated and in much pain

Pulse 120/min. BP-108/90

Weight applied to right chest area: noticeable improvement of breathing and color

5:15 P.M. Chest x-ray revealed fractures of third, fourth, and fifth ribs of left chest.

5:30 P.M. Respirations more normal; 32

Pulse 92, BP-120/80

Plan: Intubate with cuffed endotracheal tube

Positive pressure breathing through tube with volume-controlled respirator

Will suction PRN

Control pain with Meperidine.

PHYSIOLOGICAL IMPLICATIONS OF MULTIPLE RIB FRACTURES

Let's analyze this to see what caused Miss Callahan's physiological disturbances.

Paradoxical respirations

Miss Callahan had sustained a flail (unstable) chest, as a result of fractured ribs. Therefore, her chest wall rigidity on the left side

Figure 29. Left. *Normal inspiration.* Right. *Normal expiration.*

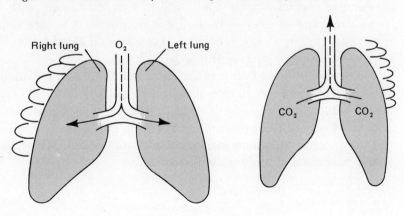

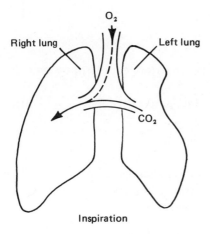
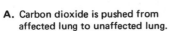
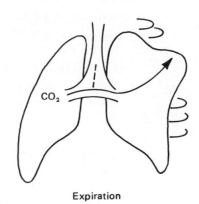

Inspiration   Expiration

A. Carbon dioxide is pushed from   **B.** Carbon dioxide is pulled into af-
affected lung to unaffected lung.   fected lung from unaffected lung.

Figure 30. *Paradoxical respirations.**
    A. *Inspiration.*
    B. *Expiration.*

of the rib-cage was lost. As a consequence, she developed a swinging, or flutter of her mediastinum and paradoxical* respirations.

On inspiration, the part of the lung underlying the fractured ribs sucked in and pushed the stale air (CO2) over into the right unaffected lung. On expiration, the weakened area on the left side bulged out and pulled the CO2 from the right lung over to the left. This swishing of carbon dioxide from lung to lung continued, with little to no exchange of oxygen from the atmosphere. A severe hypoxic state resulted; implying a deficiency of oxygenated blood to the brain, heart, and all other parts of the body.

The swinging, or flutter of the mediastinum prevented adequate venous return to the right side of the heart. Consequently, the cardiac output was decreased and reflected in a low systolic blood pressure.

Obviously, if the pressure had not been applied to the left chest wall to decrease the abnormal respiratory movement, Miss Callahan would have died of asphyxiation and shock.

* Opposite of normal.

Questions

1. Explain Miss Callahan's high diastolic pressure of 90, before treatment was instituted.
2. Explain her diastolic pressure of 80, following treatment.
3. Explain the discrepancy of her systolic pressure before and after treatment.
4. Explain the pallor and cyanosis.
5. What signs of cerebral hypoxia were present?
6. Explain her reduced pulse rate after treatment.
7. What effect does chest pain have on respirations?

REFERENCES

Beland, Irene. *Clinical Nursing,* 2nd ed. New York: Macmillan Publishing Co., Inc., 1970, p. 268.

Bordicks, Katherine J. *Nursing Care of Patients Having Chest Surgery.* New York: Macmillan Publishing Co., Inc., 1962.

Harrison's *Principles of Internal Medicine,* 8th ed. G. Thorn, R. Adams, E. Braunwald, K. Isselbacher, and R. Petersdorf, New York: McGraw-Hill Book Co., 1977, p. 1395.

Killough, John H. "Protective Mechanisms of the Lungs; Pulmonary Disease; Pleural Disease," in William A. Sodeman and William A. Sodeman, Jr. *Pathological Physiology,* 5th ed. Philadelphia: W. B. Saunders Co., 1974, pp. 393–414.

Luckmann, Joan, and Karen Sorensen. *Medical-Surgical Nursing.* Philadelphia W. B. Saunders Co., 1974.

McCredie, John A. (Ed.). *Basic Surgery.* New York: Macmillan Publishing Co., Inc., 1977.

Richardson, J. David. "Management of Noncardiac Thoracic Trauma." *Heart and Lung,* 7 (Mar.–Apr. 1978), 286–292.

Secor, Jane. *Patient Care in Respiratory Problems.* Saunders Monograph in Clinical Nursing 1. Philadelphia: W. B. Saunders Co., 1969.

Sodeman, William A., and William A. Sodeman, Jr. *Pathologic Physiology,* 5th ed. Philadelphia: W. B. Saunders Co., 1974.

"The Risk of Pneumothorax in Artificial Ventilation." *Medical World News* (June 1973), 34.

CHAPTER 12

Neurogenic Shock and
Vasogenic Shock
(Shock Due to Decreased
Vascular Tone)

Shock due to a decreased volume of blood and shock due to an inadequate heart pump have been discussed in the last two chapters. The third piece of our puzzle—the vascular tone—and different conditions affecting it which cause shock will be discussed in this chapter.

Shock represents a disproportion between the circulating blood volume and the size of the vascular bed. In health, a dynamic equilibrium is maintained between the blood volume, the heart pump mechanism, and the size of the vascular bed. This dynamic equilibrium maintains a sufficient supply of blood to all body tissues. When a threat is posed to any one of these three mechanisms, the other two, to a degree, are able to compensate for the deficiency, thereby maintaining a blood flow to body tissues sufficient to sustain life for a while.

We have seen, however, that the length of time and the degree to which the compensatory mechanisms can be sustained are limited, and, unless the deficiency or weakness is corrected, the patient cannot survive.

Neurogenic shock and vasogenic shock represent an increased size of the vascular bed—massive vasodilatation—with subsequent implications of decreased blood pressure, decreased return of venous blood to the heart, and decreased cardiac output. The overall effect is an insufficient supply of blood to body tissues; hence, a decreased supply of nutrients and oxygen to the cells, and decreased removal of cellular wastes. Tissue anoxia and cell destruction result.

In both neurogenic shock and vasogenic shock, there are an increased size of the vascular bed and a normal volume of blood. An increase in the vascular capacity, a decrease in the blood volume, or decreased heart action will reduce the mean circulatory pressure. In turn, the pressure gradient for the venous return of blood is decreased which results in a venous "pooling" of blood, a decreased venous return to the heart, and decreased cardiac output.

Although vasodilatation occurs in both neurogenic and vasogenic shock, the mechanisms producing vasodilatation in each instance are different. In neurogenic shock, the vasodilatation throughout the body is due to a diminished vasomotor tone, hence, a diminished vasoconstrictor tone; whereas in vasogenic shock the mechanism(s) causing vasodilatation in the first stage is not completely understood at present.

Neurogenic Shock

Neurogenic shock can result from any of the following:

1. Deep general anesthesia, which can depress the vasomotor center of the brain sufficiently to cause vasomotor collapse.

2. Spinal anesthesia, especially if it extends all the way up the spinal cord, the result of which is a blockage of the sympathetic nervous impulses from the nervous system. (Arterial blood pressure is reduced to 40 or 50 mm. Hg.) This is a very common cause of neurogenic shock.

3. Brain damage, such as concussions or contusions of the basal areas of the brain can cause profound neurogenic shock. Prolonged ischemia of the medulla oblongata can result in death of the vasomotor neurons; hence, the development of severe neurogenic shock.

4. Fainting caused by decreased sympathetic activity results in dilatation of the peripheral blood vessels in which the blood pools, and as a consequence the cardiac output falls drastically. Fortunately, the individual who faints falls to a horizontal position, which favors the venous return of blood to the heart and almost normal cardiac output. If the person remained in an upright position, however, the

blood would pool in the dilated peripheral vessels, with a resultant drastic reduction of venous return and cardiac output. Such an individual could go into progressive shock and die.

Let us consider a patient in neurogenic shock, as a result of spinal anesthesia.

NEUROGENIC SHOCK DUE TO SPINAL ANESTHESIA

Mr. Bill Wolfe, forty-two years of age, had a herniorrhaphy under spinal anesthesia. His normal blood pressure on admission to the hospital was 134/72 mm. Hg., and his general physical condition was good.

Postoperatively, Mr. Wolfe was receiving a pint of blood intravenously to replace blood lost in surgery. It dripped at a slow rate. His dressing was dry. During the 30 minutes after surgery, his blood pressure was checked three times and read 120/60, 114/48, and 100/26 mm. Hg. He tried to sit up but collapsed in bed as he anxiously stated how dizzy and weak he felt. His skin was pale and damp. He began to retch with nausea. His pulse rate was 80 per minute, full, and regular. (In shock due to massive vasodilatation, the mean pressure will be very low, but the pulse pressure may be greater than normal.) His respirations were increased slightly, and, as was stated, his blood pressure was markedly below his preoperative normal blood pressure. His veins were full and prominent and did not collapse when digital pressure was applied. Mr. Wolfe was in neurogenic shock.

Implications for treatment and nursing care

Unless the nurse is able to differentiate between hemorrhagic shock and neurogenic shock, she might take the wrong steps which could prove dangerous, and maybe fatal, to the patient—she might increase the rate of flow of the blood transfusion, and this certainly is not indicated in this instance. In order to solve the mystery, the nurse must use the clues she has at hand. Five clues have been given: (1) Mr. Wolfe's normal blood pressure is 134/72, (2) he had spinal anesthesia, (3) his pulse was full and regular, (4) his dressing was dry, and (5) his distended veins did not collapse on digital pressure. These clues should indicate to the nurse that Mr. Wolfe's shock is due to massive vasodilatation caused by a lack of sympathetic vasomotor innervation of his peripheral blood vessels and is not due to a decreased blood volume. Because of the effects of the spinal anesthesia, the sympathetic nerves are unable to discharge impulses to the peripheral blood vessels to constrict them. Hence, these blood vessels relax with resulting vasodilatation. This heralds in pooling of blood in the dilated vessels, decreased venous return, and decreased cardiac output. Following this, of course, is generalized tissue hypoxia along with other signs and symptoms of oxygen deficiency. (Cyanosis is rarely present in neurogenic shock. Why?) The nurse presents the facts to the physician who may prescribe a vasoconstrictor drug if the vasodilation is pronounced over an extended period of time. Usually, however, vasoconstrictors are not indicated; when the effects of the spinal anesthetic wear off, he will be able to maintain his own vasoconstriction.

Indiscriminate use of vasopressors could intensify renal vasoconstriction to the extent that ischemic nephrosis could develop, leading to oliguria or anuria. Therefore, for pulmonary and renal purposes, vasopressor therapy should be discontinued as soon as the immediate threat of shock is over. During the next few days, the volume of urine should be measured frequently (at hourly intervals, if possible). A sharp decline in renal output, in the absence of any signs of shock, could mean that ischemic nephrosis is developing. If this occurs, fluid intake and potassium are usually ordered to be limited.

If the nurse assumed that Mr. Wolfe's decreased blood pressure was due to hemorrhagic shock, and if she therefore increased the rate of the blood transfusion, she might overload his circulatory circuit which already has a sufficient volume of blood. Then, once his vasomotor tone had been restored, or had been stimulated with levarterenol drugs, the overload of circulating blood would put a burden on his heart. In the presence of any cardiac weakness, this additional burden could result in congestive heart failure and pulmonary edema, from which the patient could drown in his own blood. Therefore it is dangerous to *assume*. One must make certain, and the best way to be certain is to search for the facts and go on from there. Also, one must clearly know what to look for, and what one is likely to find. This, of course, implies that the nurse must be equipped with a body of scientific knowledge from which she can draw conclusions and base her actions. Why is a supine position indicated?

GENERAL ANESTHESIA

The development of hypotension during recovery from a general anesthetic may be due to any of the following causes:

Hemorrhage

A change in position (lithotomy to horizontal)

A change from a high to low oxygen or carbon dioxide content of inspired gas or air

Existing cardiac disease

Pain

Excessive narcosis

Blood transfusion reaction.

Inductive and deductive reasoning must be exercised. Each of the previous mentioned items must be taken into consideration in determining the cause of the particular patient's low blood pressure. To facilitate and to expedite this checking, the nurse must use the clues she has on hand.

What kind of anesthetic was administered?

Are the respiratory passages clear?

Is the patient receiving oxygen? Is it a mixture of oxygen and carbon dioxide?

Are there any signs of a transfusion reaction? Does the blood typing and the Rh factor of the blood he is receiving check with his record?

What narcotic did he have? When? How much?

Is he complaining of excessive pain?

Does he have a known cardiac weakness?

Approximately how much blood was lost during surgery?

In a word, the nurse has to be a detective, a Sherlock Holmes, as she separates the probable from the possible cause of hypotension.

INSULIN SHOCK

PRINCIPLE 49:–The metabolism of glucose in the human body (with the exception of brain tissue) is dependent on a sufficient amount of insulin in the blood stream.

Insulin shock can be classified under either cardiogenic or neurogenic categories. Because of its profound effect on the central nervous system, however, let us discuss it in the neurogenic classification.

Whereas diabetic shock is characterized by hyperglycemia which is caused by too little insulin in the body (hypoinsulinism), insulin shock is characterized by hypoglycemia, resulting from too much insulin in the body (hyperinsulinism). Both diabetic and insulin shock lurk as potential dangers to the patient who has diabetes mellitus.

Insulin regulates carbohydrate metabolism and is thought to lower the blood sugar by (1) increasing its utilization by the cells, (2) enhancing liver glycogen formation, and (3) increasing muscle glycogen formation. With an excess amount of insulin in the blood stream, a decreased blood sugar (hypoglycemia) occurs. Eventually, therefore, glucose is not available for cellular metabolism. Although the entire body is adversely affected by the lack of glucose for cellular utilization, the most vulnerable area is the central nervous system. The central nervous system essentially derives all its energy from the metabolism of glucose. Insulin is not necessary for the metabolism of glucose by the brain cells, but since increased insulin causes a decrease in blood glucose, the blood that circulates to the brain will be deficient in glucose; hence, metabolism within the central nervous system will become greatly depressed. The vasomotor system within the brain is likewise affected. As a consequence, the vasomotor nerves lose their ability to maintain the tonus of blood vessels, and the blood vessels dilate, causing hypotension.

The heart, as well as the central nervous system, is adversely affected by hyperinsulinism:

The chief signs and symptoms of insulin shock are due to the abnormally low supply of glucose to the brain cells:

1. Excitability. When the blood sugar level falls to 50 to 70 mg per cent, the hypoglycemia seems to facilitate neuronal activity.

2. Hallucinations may or may not be present.

3. Extreme nervousness and trembling. The increased irritability of the nerves that innervate the voluntary muscles causes spontaneous involuntary muscular twitchings or contractions. Patients sometimes tremble so violently that the entire bed will shake.

4. Sweating occurs due to the initial increased stimulation of the sympathetic nervous system.

5. Numbness of the lips.

6. Mental confusion ⎫
7. Faintness   ⎬ These are due to decreased metabolism within the brain.
8. Drowsiness   ⎭

9. Decreased blood pressure follows the eventual failure of the vasomotor nerves of the sympathetic nervous system to maintain vasoconstriction. The heart muscle is very dependent on glucose for its power of contraction, and when deprived of glucose, cardiac contrac-

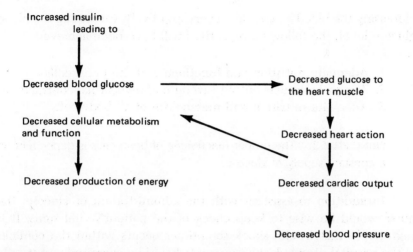

Increased insulin
    leading to

Decreased blood glucose ⟶ Decreased glucose to the heart muscle

Decreased cellular metabolism and function

Decreased heart action

Decreased production of energy

Decreased cardiac output

Decreased blood pressure

tions weaken and are followed by a decreased cardiac output and a subsequent fall in blood pressure.

10. Increased pulse rate due to the initial compensatory effects of vasoconstriction. When this fails, the pulse will feel full but weak.

11. Weakness due to the lack of glucose in the muscle cells, the stored glucose having been mobilized in an effort to increase the blood sugar, and also due to the severe involuntary muscular contractions.

12. A staggering gait and irrational hostile behavior are often misinterpreted as drunkenness.

As the blood glucose level falls to 20 to 50 mg per cent, clonic convulsions and loss of consciousness occur. With a further decrease in blood glucose, the convulsions may cease, and coma becomes manifest. Unless treatment is given immediately, permanent damage to the nerve cells of the central nervous system will take place.

Sometimes it is difficult to distinguish between diabetic shock and insulin shock. However, it must be remembered that acetone breath and rapid breathing are present in diabetic shock but not in insulin shock.

Implications for treatment and nursing care

The chief objective is to increase the blood sugar level in order to make glucose readily available for tissue use. Therefore, large quantities of glucose are given intravenously, which usually brings the patient out of shock within a minute or so. Sometimes the physician will prefer to inject epinephrine, which causes glycogenolysis in the liver, thereby increasing the blood glucose level very rapidly. By increasing the blood glucose level, the following objectives will have been achieved:

1. Adequate nutrition and functioning of the brain cells
2. Adequate cardiac output (strength of myocardial contractions)
3. Adequate nutrition and metabolism of all body cells.

PRINCIPLE 52:   The proper functioning of brain cells is dependent on a constant supply of glucose.

In addition to assisting with the administration of glucose, the nurse would be wise to keep check of the patient's vital signs. It is regrettable that insulin shock sometimes occurs within the confines of the hospital. Prophylactic measures should be exercised and strictly enforced, in order to prevent the occurrence of insulin shock. Extreme caution should be taken in measuring and checking insulin types and dosages. Errors of overdosage and the administration of the wrong type of insulin occur through carelessness, hurry, and preoccupation. Unless the nurse is alone on a service, it is always wise to double-check the following with another person:

The written order
The syringe containing the insulin
The bottle from which the insulin was withdrawn
The type of insulin
The unit of insulin must correspond to the unit side of the syringe
The time the insulin is to be given.

This double-checking process should apply not only to the student nurse but to the registered nurse as well, since all human beings are subject to committing errors.

Besides an overdosage of insulin, the patient's failure to eat his prescribed diet may also account for signs of hyperinsulinism. After every meal, his tray should be checked thoroughly, so that necessary replacements for uneaten food can be made.

In the event that signs and symptoms of hyperinsulinism do occur, the nurse must understand the physiological mechanisms involved, as well as be able to differentiate between signs and symptoms of insulin shock and diabetic shock.

Vasogenic Shock (Anaphylactic Shock and Toxic Shock)

Vasogenic shock, like neurogenic shock, is characterized by massive vasodilatation. However, the cause of the vasodilatation in each of these types of shock is different; hence, the treatment also must be different. The treatment, as we know, must be aimed toward the elimination of the factor or factors causing the vasodilatation.

Vasogenic shock is due to vasodilatation and is followed by this chain of events:

Decreased venous return
Decreased cardiac output
Decreased blood pressure
Decreased blood to body tissues
Increasing tissue anoxia and destruction

ANAPHYLACTIC SHOCK

Anaphylactic shock is due to an allergic reaction which leads to circulatory shock with a marked loss of plasma from the vascular compartment into the interstitial compartment. It is characterized by arteriolar and venous dilatation, increased capillary permeability, decreased cardiac output, and decreased systolic and diastolic blood pressure.

Miss Tena Wall, aged fifty-five years, went to the office of her dentist with complaints of a "sore gum," which was due to an infection. After he incised the gum, the dentist gave her a dose of penicillin intramuscularly. Ten minutes later, as she was putting on her coat to leave, Miss Wall became very dizzy, weak, and short of breath. She fainted. Another patient awaiting her turn shouted for the dentist. Immediately, the dentist administered epinephrine and an antihistaminic drug intravenously. Within a half minute, Miss Wall regained consciousness and, looking up at the dentist, asked, "What happened?" Replied the dentist, "You passed out, Miss Wall. I think you're allergic to penicillin. Just rest on the couch for a while. You'll feel all right soon."

ALLERGIC REACTIONS TO DRUGS

Allergy, or hypersensitivity, implies an altered reactivity to a foreign substance as a result of previous contact with it. Interestingly enough, this violent antigen-antibody reaction does not occur after the first exposure to the antigen; it occurs after the second exposure. And why it occurs in some individuals and not in others is unknown. (Could our genetic patterns be one possible answer?)

In anaphylactic shock, a violent antigen-antibody reaction is the cause of severe and even fatal symptoms. Allergic reactions to drugs are becoming more prevalent. It is generally believed that allergic reactions are due to harmful immune reactions. Drug allergy can be manifested dermatologically and/or systemically. The symptoms usually appear during the second week of therapy, or after the second dosage of the drug, or even after a longer time interval at which time the individual is treated with the drug for the second time. In the time interval between the first and second encounter with the drug, the body develops antibodies to the drug antigens. The reaction between these antibodies and the newly injected or ingested antigens can cause a harmful immune reaction which, if violent enough, will result in anaphylactic shock. In our example of Miss Wall, the drug causing her state of shock was penicillin. However, it should be stated at this time that the drug doesn't exist that someone isn't allergic to—and this includes aspirin. Individuals are also allergic to foods, pollens, smoke, cat hair, paint, wool, and so on. If the reaction to any of these is sufficiently violent, anaphylactic shock can result.

Allergic reactions and diseases are poorly understood. Individuals who are allergic (hypersensitive) react in a violent or unusual manner to foreign substances (antigens) that produce little or no reaction in others.

The major symptoms resulting from the abnormal cellular release of histamine and other kinins (bradykinin, serotonin, S-R* substance) into the blood stream are the following:

> Anxiety
> Severe dyspnea—cyanosis
> Marked edema of face, hands, or general edema
> Itching
> Diffuse erythema
> Abdominal cramps
> Vomiting and/or diarrhea
> Unconsciousness.

* Slow reacting substance.

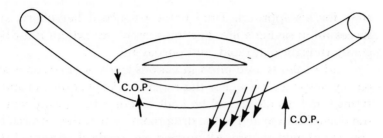

Figure 31. *Excessive loss of fluid from the intravascular compartment.*

Unless appropriate treatment is given immediately, death can ensue rapidly.

PHYSIOLOGICAL IMPLICATIONS OF ANAPHYLACTIC SHOCK

In anaphylactic shock, the following occur:

1. Arteriolar and venous dilatation.
2. Increased capillary permeability.

As a result, there is a marked abnormal shift of fluid into the interstitial compartment, thus decreasing the circulating blood volume. This results in a decreased venous return and decreased cardiac output, decreased systolic and diastolic blood pressure, and generalized edema.

3. Intense bronchiolar constriction leading to a generalized hypoxic state.

Implications for treatment and nursing care

OBJECTIVE 1: Facilitate the respiratory exchange of oxygen and carbon dioxide.

Immediate treatment calls for the administration of adrenalin to dilate the bronchioles. This is the chief priority. Oxygen, antihistaminics, and vasoconstrictors are also usually indicated. Adrenalin should be readily available for emergency use. Loss of a few minutes in obtaining the drug, syringe, and needle may be responsible for the death of the individual. Adrenalin can be given subcutaneously by the nurse, or intravenously by the physician. Although the nurse does not prescribe the medication to be given, she must be able to recognize the indications for such a medication, and to contact the physician immediately for his approval. Time is the essence if her efforts are to be successful in saving a life. For this reason, her actions must be intelligently thought out, rapid, and purposeful.

Adrenalin is used often in various kinds of emergency situations on any hospital service. For this reason, a vial of adrenalin and a sterile syringe and needle should be kept together in a prominent place in the nurses' station and in the drug room, so that they are readily available for immediate use. All nursing and medical personnel should be informed of this location. Valuable minutes can be lost in searching through a box containing an assortment of emergency drugs. Indeed, such boxes often defeat the purpose for which they are intended.

An allergic condition represents stress, which causes an increased secretion of glucocorticoids into the blood stream. This is a favorable response, because glucocorticoids help the body resist cellular damage, reduce the severity of allergic reactions, and also prevent inflammation of damaged and diseased tissues. It is thought that glucocorticoids tend to reduce the formation of cellular proteins, such as immune bodies, that are responsible for either allergic or inflammatory reactions. Very large doses reduce and sometimes completely block antibody formation. Glucocorticoids may be prescribed for this patient, in order to supplement her own secretion of them.

OBJECTIVE 2.   Improve patient's circulatory status.

Remobilization of fluid from the interstitial compartment back into the vascular compartment is indicated. It's obvious that, in order to restore normal circulatory dynamics, the blood vessels must be constricted to a more normal size. A vasoconstrictor drug is usually indicated.

The patient should be placed in a supine position to facilitate the flow of blood to the brain.

OBJECTIVE 3:   Help to prevent future allergic attacks.
PRINCIPLE 60:   Means are taken for protection and defense when an enemy is known.
PRINCIPLE 61:   Forewarning predisposes to forearming.
PRINCIPLE 62:   Human beings have a right to know those things that concern them.
PRINCIPLE 63:   Protection of self is a responsibility and a right.

The drug to which the patient is allergic usually is discontinued. The nurse must make sure that the medication card is destroyed, and that notification of the patient's allergy to the particular drug is clearly made on the patient's chart and cardex, preferably on the front cover of the chart, so that it can be seen by all who read the chart. If future episodes of anaphylactic shock are to be avoided, the patient must be informed of the particular drug to which he is allergic. In turn, the patient should notify his family physician and dentist of this. If he enters a hospital as a patient, he should, on admission, notify his attending head nurse and physician of his allergy, so that he is not given this drug in his treatment. Because of the possibility that the patient might forget the name of the drug, it should be written on a piece of paper for him. It might also be suggested that the patient secure a meditag, or bracelet which is engraved: "I am allergic to penicillin," or whatever drug may be involved. This is also a good suggestion for diabetics and cardiac patients.

Because of the increasing incidence of drug allergies, it is becoming common practice in many hospitals to tell the patient the names of drugs he is receiving. This is very good practice. It has often happened that on being informed of the name of the drug about to be administered, the patient spoke up and said, "Oh, I can't take that drug. I'm allergic to it." Thus, anaphylactic shock and possibly death may have been prevented. Aside from the risk of allergy, why shouldn't people be told the names of drugs they are expected to swallow or take by injection? It concerns *them!* As individuals in a free society, persons have a basic right to know those things which concern them!

TOXIC SHOCK (SYNONYMS: SEPTIC SHOCK, BACTERIAL SHOCK, BACTEREMIC SHOCK, ENDOTOXIC SHOCK)

Comparison with other types of shock
In shock due to myocardial infarction the cardiac output is low, and the vascular resistance may be normal to high. In shock due to the loss of blood the cardiac output is low and the vascular resistance is high. In the initial phase of shock due to toxins, however, the cardiac output is high and the vascular resistance is low.

Causes of toxic shock
Toxic shock can be produced by two toxins: (1) exotoxins, and (2) endotoxins. These toxins are breakdown products of bacteria. To date, little is known about the effects produced by exotoxins, and there is much more to be learned about the nature of endotoxins. We do

know, however, that endotoxins are intense vasoconstrictors. This occurs in the last, or "cold" phase of toxic shock.

Toxic shock has a high mortality and remains incompletely understood. Studies of the toxic shock syndrome in man have failed to separate the effects of sepsis from the effects of the patients' underlying disease. Toxic shock can be due to a wide variety of organisms, e.g., endotoxic shock is due to Gram negative bacteria, such as Escherichia coli, Airobacter-Klebsiella, Proteus mirabilis or vulgaris, and Pseudomonas aerugenosa. Other organisms are Paracolon bacilli, Salmonella, Coliform organisms, and so on.

GRAM NEGATIVE SHOCK

Shock due to Gram negative enteric bacteria is believed to be a common complication of a select type of bacterial infection invading the blood stream. More commonly, it occurs in the older person and in pregnant women and is often mistaken for myocardial infarction. Pregnant women with toxic shock are considered high-risk patients. This type of shock can be due to infected abortions, pyleonephritis during pregnancy,* and chorioaminionitis. Recovery of these patients is achieved only by prompt diagnosis and aggressive management.

INCIDENCE OF TOXIC SHOCK

Other than in pregnant women, toxic shock is rarely seen in persons under forty years of age. The median age is sixty, and it occurs twice as frequently in men as in women.

Toxic shock occurs most frequently in patients with urinary tract infections which are often precipitated by manipulative† or surgical procedures involving the urinary tract, pelvis, or perineum in the presence of infection.

It is believed that antibiotics given for Gram *positive* infections cause an increase in certain Gram negative infections, and hence an increase in bacteremia and shock.

---

* In the pregnant woman, toxic shock due to pyleonephritis, is partially the result of urinary stasis due to mechanical pressure on the ureters by the uterus. The patient should be instructed to lie on her side to relieve the pressure and hence improve urinary flow.

† Catheters, sounds, and cystoscopes are examples of precipitating agents.

OTHER MAJOR SOURCES OF BACTEREMIC INFECTION

Other sources of bacteremic infection are

1. The intestinal flora, lower ileum and colon, biliary tract, chole-cystitis, subphrenic abscess associated with duodenal perforation, intra-abdominal abscesses, peritonitis, cirrhosis and ascites, and penetrating abdominal trauma.
2. Female genital tract: septic abortion, pelvic inflammatory disease, pelvic abscess, and postgynecologic surgery.
3. Lower respiratory tract: pneumonitis, necrotizing pneumonia, aspiration pneumonia, respiratory and tracheostomy-induced.
4. Meningitis.
5. Skin and soft tissue abscesses, cellulitis, decubitus ulcers.
6. Toxins may enter the blood stream in the following situations:
   a. Thrombosis of the intestinal arteries. Toxins formed by bacteria in the gangrenous intestine can cause profound shock.
   b. If tourniquets are applied too tightly over a prolonged period of time. A tourniquet should be tightened sufficiently to cause venous congestion in the extremity without obliterating the arterial pulse, and hence the obliteration of arterial blood to the extremity. The arterial pulse point below the applied tourniquet should be checked frequently. No extremity should be compressed longer than sixty minutes at any one time; and no less than five minutes should intervene between successive compressions of the same limb. In addition to the entrance of toxins into the blood stream, if a tourniquet is applied too tightly, or over a lengthy period of time, phlebothrombosis and/or fatal pulmonary embolism could occur.
7. Severe burns: Toxic factors from damaged tissues, including considerable amounts of histamine, serotonin, and bradykinin can make the burn shock more pronounced.

UNDERLYING PHYSIOLOGICAL MECHANISM?

In the past, the underlying physiological mechanism causing toxic shock was believed to have been vasomotor collapse, which is characterized by marked arteriolar dilatation. Later, it was thought that the toxic shock mechanism was due to a generalized injury to the heart and peripheral vessels.

261

More recently, it has been suggested that vascular occlusion by multiple blood clots is implicated in the disease, which leads to ischemic injury. The question of the underlying mechanism remains unresolved. Perhaps posterity will divulge the answer to this question.

THE TRAUMA PATIENT AND TOXIC SHOCK

The patient with trauma who develops toxic shock with multiple organ failure is very likely to die. Multiple systems insufficiency is a sequence of organ failures. Pulmonary failure usually occurs first. Right ventricular failure, secondary to elevated pulmonary vascular resistance, usually occurs next. This is followed by liver failure, which is evidenced by jaundice and hypoalbuminemia. Typically, the occurrence of these failures is within seven to fourteen days post trauma. If terminal, a deficiency of most clotting factors occurs, and the patient is likely to die of hemorrhagic shock.

The two phases of toxic shock

There is general agreement among the authorities that toxic shock consists of two phases: the early, or "warm" phase, and the late, or "cold" phase.

The early ("warm") phase. The following occur:

1. Vasodilatation—flushed face, warm skin, decreasing diastolic BP. Due to the release of vasoactive substances, such as histamine.
2. Temperature usually over 102 degrees Fahrenheit. A shaking chill may coincide with temperature peaks.
3. Alert—suggesting sufficient blood-flow to the brain; hence, we know that the venous return is satisfactory at this time. Apprehension may or may not be present.
4. Increased cardiac output and increased stroke volume. Pulse pressure within a satisfactory range. Urinary output satisfactory.
5. Moderate tachycardia (100–120 per minute). Approximately 20 per cent of the patients have a pulse rate of 72 or less per minute.
6. Gradual reduction in venous return, leading to a gradual reduction in cardiac output; therefore, a decreasing systolic BP. It is believed that the venules are constricted at this time, and

the arterioles are relaxed, dilated. This may be the result of histamine-release; when present in large amounts, histamine constricts venules and dilates arterioles. Therefore, with decreased arteriolar resistance, there is an increase in capillary pressure, and large amounts of plasma fluid enter the interstitial compartment. Also, an increased venous resistance leads to an increased capillary pressure, preventing the exit of fluid from the interstitial compartment. It has also been postulated that the decline in cardiac output may be due to a specific myocardial depressant factor (MDF).

7. Metabolic alkalosis due to hyperventilation.

The late (cold) phase

1. Extreme vasoconstriction—presumably due to endotoxins and extreme sympathetic nervous system hyperactivity (a latent effect?) with increases of epinephrine and norepinephrine. Released from the cells (as a result of the toxic insult) are histamine, serotonin, bradykinin, kallikren II, and angiotensin II.

2. Cold, pale skin (due to arteriolar constriction), and clammy skin (due to the increased sympathetic activity).

3. Subnormal temperature (heat having been dissipated as a result of the warm phase?). Low body temperature is an indication of the inability of the body to maintain metabolic heat production sufficient to offset the heat loss.

4. Decreased venous return, due to venous constriction. Decreased cardiac output, decreased stroke volume.

5. Oliguria, due to decreased GFR, and renal arteriolar vasoconstriction.

6. Patient gradually becomes less alert. Often, the first indication of a hypotensive state is an alteration in the patient's mental status; the speech becomes incoherent, the behavior is inappropriate, and the patient becomes confused and stuporous.

7. Disseminated intravascular clotting (DIC)—a sludging of blood in the vessels. This leads to decreased tissue perfusion and dangers of emboli.

8. Metabolic acidosis. Cell hypoxia leads to anaerobic metabolism and metabolic acidosis.

9. Anuria. The second most common cause of death in toxic shock is acute or chronic renal failure.

10. Coma, suggesting decreased blood to the brain.
11. Cardiac and respiratory distress. Most deaths from toxic shock are due to the "shock-lung syndrome."

EFFECTS OF TOXIC SHOCK ON THE BODY

Although the underlying mechanism of toxic shock has not been identified, we do know some of the major deleterious effects of toxic shock on the body. These are:

1. Impaired kidney function due to intense renal vasoconstriction. This leads to an increased release of renin from the ischemic kidney, which in turn increases the amount of angiotensin in the blood. Angiotensin stimulates the release of aldosterone which conserves sodium, and hence water, and it also is a potent vasoconstrictor.
2. Increased alveolocapillary permeability leads to pulmonary insufficiency which leads to the shock-lung syndrome.
3. Heart failure, after six or nine hours.
4. Inadequate perfusion of blood in various body organs.
5. D.I.C. The endotoxins activate the clotting mechanism. Numerous clots plug small peripheral vessels.
6. Capillary damage leading to increased capillary permeability. Increased loss of fluids into the interstitial compartment, decreased venous return, decreased cardiac output, decreasing systolic BP.
7. Metabolic acidosis accentuates blood clotting.

THE DIAGNOSIS AND TREATMENT OF TOXIC SHOCK

Toxic shock is diagnosed only when a blood or wound culture reveals the causative organism. Antibiotic sensitivity testing must be done. Treatment may be medical or surgical, or both.

1. An adequate airway must be maintained. An endotracheal tube, or a tracheostomy may be necessary. Suctioning is usually indicated. Incision and drainage of localized collection of pus should be done, and is usually indicated.
2. Antibiotic therapy should be prompt and based upon the microscopic results of the smear. If Pseudomonas is present, Gentamycin is presently the antibiotic of choice.

3. Other drugs which may be indicated are
   a. Glucocorticoids—presumably because of their anti-inflammatory effects in decreasing capillary permeability. Corticoids oppose the vasodilatation caused by bradykinin and histamine.
   b. Vasopressor drug therapy—to improve tissue-perfusion, rather than to restore a "normal" BP. If, while in the "warm" phase of shock (characterized by vasodilatation), a vasopressor is given, it will improve the BP that will ensure an adequate coronary blood flow and urine output. During the "cold" phase (characterized by vasoconstriction), a vasodilator plus volume-replacement with a plasma-expander may be indicated.
   c. Dopamine, an inotropic agent to increase myocardial contractility without excessive peripheral vasoconstriction. Dopamine also dilates the mesenteric and renal vascular beds, thus ensuring adequate circulation to these parts and decreasing the tendency for clot formation in these vessels.
   d. Digitalis for improved cardiac performance.
   e. Heparin to control clotting.
4. Fluid-volume and electrolyte replacement—plasma volume expanders such as albumin and amino acids are usually more effective if given early. The septic patient needs far greater quantities of these than is required in health to maintain a normal plasma albumin. The CVP, PAWP, and urinary output should be monitored to detect any signs of fluid-overload, a sign of heart failure. When the colloid osmotic pressure is improved, urinary output usually increases and is followed by a decreased pulmonary capillary alveolar extravasation. If shock lung is present, with a high CVP and PWP, colloids are usually required to decrease the pulmonary congestion. Lactic acids, arterial blood gases, and pH serve as guides in the replacement of potassium and in the management of acidosis. Patients in septic shock may be in one of three acid/base imbalances: respiratory alkalosis, compensated metabolic acidosis, or decompensated metabolic acidosis.
5. Hypothermia—Engle and Rink's experiments of hypothermia on rats have suggested that this may buy time for aggressive alternate therapy in instances of toxic shock. Hypothermia, when used during the warm, or early phase of toxic shock,

reduces the metabolic demands of the body. Therefore, there is an alleviation of tachycardia, protecting cardiac energy stores; the blood glucose level is sustained; there is an increase in the $pO2$ due to increasing solubility of oxygen in plasma with decreasing temperatures; and there is a decreased need for oxygen by the tissues, thereby decreasing tissue blood flow.[1]

IMPLICATIONS FOR PREVENTION AND CONTROL
OF TOXIC SHOCK

Although toxic shock is often due to the underlying disease condition, the following can also be involved in its occurrence.

Toxic shock can result from poor technique in the cleansing and dressing of wounds. It can also result from a long-standing indwelling catheter which creates a favorable environment for infection of the bladder and/or urethra.

Contaminated monitoring devices are a source of bacterial, fungal, and viral organisms. Transducers should be cleaned with soap and water, rinsed, then sterilized between use with different patients.

Probably the most basic factor in the prevention and control of toxic shock is frequent and thorough handwashing with soap and water, before and after the care of each patient. HARMFUL ORGANISMS are spread more by the HANDS than by any other means!

Dressings are best done with sterile instruments, as the wearing of gloves gives one a sense of false security, and the gloves can easily be contaminated. There is a much greater tendency of contaminating gloves than there is in contaminating instruments. Contaminated dressings are best not touched with instruments *or* gloves. Simply putting one's hand in a plastic bag, grasping the dressing, and inverting the bag will secure the dressing in an air-tight container. The end of the bag should then be twisted and secured with a tie. Not only will this protect the person doing the dressing, but it will decrease the spread of air-borne infections to patients and personnel.

Draining wounds should be cleansed with soap and water. It is *not* sufficient to cleanse only *around* a draining wound; purulent material from the wound must be *eliminated* and the wound should be cleansed. If this is not done, there is *no* possibility that the wound would heal.

[1] Engle, Richard L., and Richard D. Rink, "Prolonged Moderate Hypothermia and Experimental Endotoxin Shock," *Journal of Surgical Research*, 21 (July 16, 1976), 7–14.

Suctioning of the airway, including suctioning through endotracheal tubes and tracheostomy tubes, should be done only under sterile technique. Sterile gloves should be worn and a sterile catheter should be used *each time* the patient is suctioned.

Implications for nursing care

Before and during the first phase (warm phase), the following objectives are indicated.

OBJECTIVE 1:   Observe patients who may be predisposed to developing toxic shock.

Intelligent observation implies that we know what we're looking for, and, to a certain extent, what we are likely to find.

OBJECTIVE 2:   Assess patient's circulatory status.

Nursing Care:

1. Monitor vital signs every 15 minutes.
    a. Compare blood pressure with normal blood pressure, if known, and report any discrepancies. In toxic shock, the diastolic pressure will decrease more rapidly than the systolic pressure, during the warm phase.
    b. Check the pulse pressure. If the diastolic pressure is decreased more than the systolic pressure, the pulse pressure will be widened.
    c. Check the temperature. An elevated temperature with alternating chills usually indicates a blood stream infection. Check skin for excessive warmth and flushing.
    d. Assess mental acuity and any apprehension or change in behavior. Place in a recumbent position to ensure an adequate flow of blood to the brain.
    e. Measure intake and output every hour.

OBJECTIVE 3:   Assess patient's respiratory status.

1. Count the respiratory rate per minute. Hyperventilation can lead to alkalosis. Observe for any signs of tetany or staring aimlessly into space, which often indicates an alkalotic condition.

An alert and knowledgeable nurse will most likely observe any alterations from normal.

267

During the second phase (cold phase), the following objectives are indicated:

OBJECTIVE 1:   Ensure an adequate supply of blood to the brain.

Nursing Care:

1. Place patient in a supine position. If the patient is pregnant, place her on her side.
2. Check mental acuity and signs of apprehension and behavior changes.

OBJECTIVE 2:   Assess general circulatory status.

Nursing Care:

1. Feel skin for degrees of coldness and clamminess. (Use backs of fingers for greater accuracy.)
2. Observe skin for pallor, which would indicate peripheral arteriolar vasoconstriction.
3. Measure intake and output every hour. (If the systolic pressure decreases, the blood flow to the kidneys will be reduced; therefore urine production will be reduced.)
4. Check the vital signs:
   a. Temperature. A subnormal temperature is typical during the cold phase.
   b. Blood pressure. Look for a decreasing systolic pressure and an increasing diastolic pressure. The pulse pressure would be narrow.
   c. Check the central venous pressure and/or the pulmonary artery wedge pressure. A rising CVP indicates a relative failure of the right side of the heart, while a rising PAWP indicates a relative failure of the left heart. Observe the neck veins for distention.
   d. Check quality and rate of the pulse. Note any indications of pulse weakness and/or irregularities.
   e. Count the respirations per minute. Observe for depth of respirations. Auscultate the chest for signs of rales, wheezing, or rhonchi.

OBJECTIVE 3:   Assess respiratory status.
OBJECTIVE 4:   Provide for adequate exchange of respiratory gases.

Nursing Care:

1. Auscultate the chest. Wet breathing usually indicates obstructed breathing. Bronchiolar constriction causes wheezing.
2. Check respiratory rate and depth.
3. Suction as needed, using sterile technique.

Record and report any abnormalities. The sooner the physician knows of any adverse findings, the sooner therapy can be started.

REFERENCES

Altura, B. M., E. E. Kobold, R. Lovell, W. Katz, and A. P. Thal. "Role of Glucocorticoids in Local Regulation of Blood Flow." *American Journal of Physiology*, **211** (1966), p. 119.

Bartlett, J., and S. Gorbach. "Antibiotic Therapy of Shock," in William Schumar and Lloyd Nyhus (Eds.). *Treatment of Shock*. Philadelphia: Lea and Febiger, 1974, pp. 157–159.

Border, J. R., R. Chenier, R. H. McMenamy, J. LaDuca, R. Seibel, R. Birkhahn, and L. Yu. "Multiple Systems Organ Failure: Muscle Fuel Deficit with Visceral Protein Malnutrition." *Surgical Clinics of North America*, **56** (Oct. 1976), 1147–1167.

Cavanagh, Denis, and Manuel R. Comas. "Management of the Patient in Septic Shock," D. Cavanagh, P. Rao, and M. Comas, *Septic Shock in Obstetrics and Gynecology*, Vol. 11 in series: Major Problems in Obstetrics and Gynecology. Consulting Ed., Emanuel A. Friedman. Philadelphia: W. B. Saunders Co., pp. 94–108.

Coleman, B. D. "Septic Shock in Pregnancy." *Obstet. Gynecology*, **24:** (1964), 895.

"Chemical Mediators Released by Endotoxin." *Surgical Gynecology, Obstetrics*, **118** (1964), 807.

Guyton, Arthur C. *Textbook of Medical Physiology*, 5th ed., Philadelphia: W. B. Saunders Co., 1976.

Harrison's *Principles of Internal Medicine*, 8th ed. G. Thorne, R. Adams, E. Braumwald, K. Isselbacher, and R. Petersdorf. New York: McGraw-Hill Book Co., 1977.

Mikal, Stanley. *Homeostasis in Man*. Boston: Little, Brown and Company, 1967, p. 482.

Sodeman, William A., and William A. Sodeman, Jr. *Pathologic Physiology*, 5th ed. Philadelphia: W. B. Saunders Co., 1974.

Weil, Max H., and Herbert Shubin. "Shock Associated with Infection—Bacterial Shock," *Diagnosis and Treatment of Shock*, Baltimore: Williams Wilkins Co., 1967, pp. 156–170.

Weinstein, R., W. Stamm, L. Kramer, and L. Corey. "Pressure Monitoring

Devices Overlooked Source of Nosocomial Infection." *Journal of the American Medical Association,* **236** (Aug. 23, 1976), 936–938.

Winslow, E., H. Loeb, S. Rahimtoola, S. Kamath, and R. Gunnar. "Hemodynamic Studies and Results of Therapy in 50 Patients With Bacteremic Shock." *The American Journal of Medicine,* **54** (Apr. 1973), 421–432.

CHAPTER 13

Conclusion

Throughout this text the different degrees of shock have been discussed. It is well to keep in mind that the patient can range from a state of full consciousness to the opposite extreme of total unconsciousness. The span between these represents degrees of semiconsciousness.

Shock represents a stress situation. The sympathetic nervous system, therefore, is hyperactive. As a result of this hyperactivity, the sensorium is more acute. Although it is important that we are always mindful of what we say in the presence of all patients, it is especially important that we choose our words carefully when we converse near the patient who is not completely conscious, including patients coming out of anesthesia and all other conditions accompanied by degrees of unconsciousness.

It is difficult to assess at what time the reversal from unconsciousness to consciousness takes place. We know that the provision of proper treatment and nursing care will start this reversal. It is also known that a seemingly unconscious patient may be in a more conscious state than we realize, despite his inability to respond to us. After their recovery, I have queried patients as to how they felt during the crucial period when they were in shock. Although some did not remember anything that occurred, many others did. Following are examples of patient's remarks: "I completely lost two whole days. I don't remember anything." "I know I was hemorrhaging. I heard the doctors and nurses talking. One doctor said, 'This is a fight against time. If we don't take her to surgery and stop this bleeding, she'll be a goner.'" One patient stated that she was too weak to open her eyes; however, she remembers hoping that her husband would remarry so that the children would be taken care of. This suggests cerebral activity, despite a profound lack of blood to that area.

Others in semiconscious, or seemingly unconscious, states have remarked about their reaction to sounds and voices. They had exaggerated reactions to loud voices, which were a source of irritation and discomfort. Soft voices, on the other hand, had the opposite effect and soothed the patient into a state of mental ease.

Besides the effect of the quality of sound, patients in semiconscious states often remember the content of what was said. But what is heard by the patient is often distorted out of all proportion by him at that particular time. Later, in convalescence, the patient can look back at his distorted reactions and perhaps smile. At the time of semiconsciousness, however, the patient is not amused. His reaction is often fear. Fear superimposed on existing apprehension is entirely out of order. It is our responsibility to allay fears and not to add to them.

In a word, we must not assume that a semiconscious, or an unconscious patient cannot hear what we say. Moreover, we must remember that if the patient hears what we say, there is a strong possibility that he will distort our meaning. For this reason, we must use extreme caution in what we say and how we say it. Even though the patient may be too weak to communicate with us, many times we are able to communicate with him. This must be shared with personnel and the patient's visitors, who might inadvertently assume that the unconscious patient cannot hear. Unhurried speaking, directed to the patient, should always be positive in nature.

Sympathy and Compassion

Sympathy and compassion for patients represent the core of humanized nursing. A proper balance between feeling and know-how is requisite in the nursing care of all patients. On the other hand, an imbalance

272

of these two factors could easily upset the emotional and physiologic being of the patient.

Although nursing care given to patients in shock is almost always of an emergency nature, requiring quick thinking and action of the nurse to provide for the patient's physiologic needs, at no time is it justifiable for the nurse to remain completely detached from the emotional needs of her patients. Although the principle, "We reassure patients mainly by what we do, rather than by what we say," is applicable to the patient whose life is severely threatened by certain physiologic needs, this does not suggest that the nurse should remain aloof and detached from the patient and his emotional needs. Indeed, while we are checking his vital signs, we have a golden opportunity to communicate warmth and compassion to him through two important senses—touch and hearing—and thereby give emotional support. Not any voice or any touch can relieve patients' apprehension. It is the voice and touch of a sincere, warmhearted, human, sympathetic person that help to relieve apprehension. In fact, much emotional support is nonverbal—the eyes and the touch do much more than is realized. The manner in which we do things for patients or assist them—the act of smiling, wiping the brow, fluffing the pillow, touching the hand— is how sympathetic understanding and compassion can be conveyed.

In her excellent article entitled "What's Wrong With Sympathy?" Joyce Travelbee says:

> Sympathy is not the same as being courteous; it is more than that. Nurses can be courteous, just as they can express pity, in a frightening, dehumanized manner that conveys neither warmth nor understanding. Sympathy is warmth and kindness, a specific expression of compassion, a caring quality experienced on a feeling level and communicated by one human being to another. It cannot be feigned despite the most elaborate communication techniques. . . .
>
> In the simplest terms, sympathy means that she cares. And in and through that caring, she can give what we call emotional support, can sustain another human being in this time of crisis. The sympathetic nurse is an authentic human being. Lacking sympathy, the nurse is a dehumanized abstraction communicating with other abstractions called "patients," and nursing becomes thereby a mechanical, dehumanized process.[1]

Although methods of communication and courtesy can be taught to nurses and learned by them, sympathetic understanding and com-

[1] Joyce Travelbee, "What's Wrong With Sympathy?" *Amer. J. Nursing,* **64** (1964), 70–71.

passion cannot be taught in a classroom. These seem to be qualities which are inherent. A nurse can learn that she is supposed to care, but whether or not she does care is quite a different matter.

There is a danger that this chapter might be misinterpreted and taken out of context. The whole of nursing care consists of a balance between the satisfaction of physiologic and emotional needs. In some patients this may mean placing more emphasis on one aspect than on the other. Each patient situation must be weighed carefully. Holding the hand of the apprehensive patient (who, in all probability, will die unless his physiologic needs are taken care of) without due regard for his physiologic needs is such an imbalance. Knowledge and judgment must be utilized at all times, if the nursing care needs of each patient are to be completely satisfied.

Finally, it is hoped that my Common Denominator Theory has been exemplified throughout this book.

When one can grasp the elements which are in common to most disease conditions, and superimpose the specific knowledge of a disease in question, one's understanding should improve remarkably. Only through improved understanding can patients receive improved nursing care.

INDEX

Principles related to the nursing care of patients in shock

30. Adequate circulation of blood to all body parts is dependent upon a proportionate equilibrium between the blood volume, the strength of cardiac contractions, and the size of the lumina of the vascular bed. 120

31. The survival of brain cells is dependent on a continuous supply of oxygen and nutrients. 160

32. Increased specialization of a unit is accompanied by increased vulnerability of that unit. 160

33. The preservation of a vital part should have precedence over the preservation of less vital parts, even at the expense of the less vital parts. 160

34. Fluids and gases flow from greater to lesser points of pressure. 160,225,235

35. Oxygen is necessary to sustain life. 162

36. The passage of oxygen from the atmosphere to the lungs, and the passage of carbon dioxide from the blood stream to the atmosphere are dependent on an open airway. 162,225

37. Every living organism is provided with a means to protect itself. 164

38. The length of time and the degree to which self-protection can be maintained are variable in different individuals. 164

39. There is a relative proportion between cellular activity and cellular requirements for oxygen and nutrients (blood):
a. Increased cellular activity (metabolism) implies an increased need for oxygen and nutrients.
b. Decreased cellular activity implies a decreased need for oxygen and nutrients. 164

40. Pain intensifies shock. 166

41. Anything that can affect man may influence his tolerance to pain. 166